Assessment for Everyone

Modifying NASPE Assessments to Include All Elementary School Children

Ellen M. Kowalski, Ph.D.
Adelphi University
Long Island, N.Y.

Lauren J. Lieberman, Ph.D.
The College at Brockport, State University of New York
Brockport, N.Y.

W9-AHB-801

Contributing Editor
Jacalyn Lea Lund, Ph.D.
Georgia State University
Atlanta, Ga.

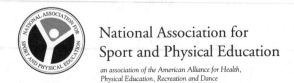

National Association for
Sport and Physical Education
an association of the American Alliance for Health,
Physical Education, Recreation and Dance

NASPE Sets the Standard

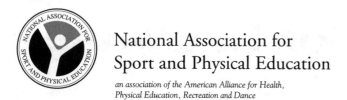

National Association for
Sport and Physical Education
*an association of the American Alliance for Health,
Physical Education, Recreation and Dance*

NASPE Sets the Standard

To order more copies of this book (stock # 304-10492):
Web: www.naspeinfo.org
E-mail: customerservice@aahperd.org
Phone: (800) 321-0789; (412) 741-1288 outside the United States
Fax: (412) 741-0609
Mail: AAHPERD Publications Fulfillment Center
            P.O. Box 1020
            Sewickley, PA 15143-1020

ISBN: 978-0-88314-950-8

Printed in the United States

Suggested citation for this book:

Lieberman, L., Kowalski, E., et al. (2011). Assessment for everyone: Modifying NASPE
assessments to include all elementary school children. Reston, VA: National Association
for Sport and Physical Education.

Contents

Preface

Because 90 percent of all students with disabilities now are included in general physical education classes, the responsibility for assessing, planning and instructing students with disabilities lies more heavily than ever with general physical education teachers. General physical educators also are becoming more involved in assessment as part of the individualized education program (IEP) process for students with disabilities.

Assessment is difficult enough for physical educators to complete in an active and dynamic setting for students *without* disabilities. To add to the challenge, many assessments that are available to teachers don't provide options for accommodating students who are low-skilled and students with disabilities within the assessment process. Using options within an assessment tool allows teachers and school districts to evaluate program success for children of all ability levels and *encourages* inclusion, indicating clearly that students with disabilities are to be part of the assessment process. Many of the existing assessments, however, don't offer ideas for including the wide range of abilities found in students today, including those with disabilities. Just as teachers modify activities to meet students' needs, so too must programmatic assessment be modified to accommodate students with disabilities.

This book expands upon assessment techniques featured in selected books with the National Association for Sport and Physical Education's (NASPE) Assessment Series to ensure that physical education teachers can assess all students — including those with disabilities — in a variety of ways. As such, this resource is designed to assist general physical educators who might not be clear about how to modify assessment protocols for children who are more difficult to reach. It will help physical educators create true instruction alignment, allowing them to determine each student's abilities and develop the appropriate instruction. Because NASPE's Assessment Series is so vast, the authors of this book have chosen ideas from only the Assessment books geared toward the elementary grades.

The format of this book is different from other books. The intent is for teachers to use the book as a helpful reference for assessment ideas presented in selected NASPE Assessment Series books that already might be in use. It is *not* necessary, however, to have the NASPE Assessment Series books to use the ideas in *this* book. Each chapter provides ideas for modifying existing assessment protocols and material found in the corresponding NASPE Assessment Series book, including the assessment environment; instruction strategies; equipment; and distances, times and set-up. Each chapter offers modifications — when appropriate — to help teachers use the NASPE assessments for students with a variety of needs, including students with physical disabilities, cognitive disabilities, sensory impairments, learning disabilities, autism spectrum disorders and emotional disorders.

Please note that these modifications are not only for students with disabilities; they are intended for any student who cannot be assessed at the level presented in each of the NASPE Assessment Series books. Those include students with low skill or fitness levels, English-as-a-second-language (ESL) students and those from culturally diverse populations that might not have had experience in that particular activity.

This is not to suggest that teachers should administer the modified assessments in isolation; instead, they should allow students of all abilities to be assessed alongside their peers.

Another difference of note is the use of Universal Design for Learning (UDL) approach in each chapter. The concept and principles of UDL, currently being applied in a variety of contexts, are explained in the first chapter, but UDL also is used in subsequent chapters as an approach for assessing students in the activities covered in those chapters.

Here is a brief outline of each chapter:

Chapter 1, Applying the Universal Design for Learning Approach to Assessment, provides an overview of UDL and how to incorporate it within assessments.

Chapter 2, Assessing Elementary Motor Skills, provides tips for modifying teacher observation checklists and cues, as well as student self-assessments so that students with disabilities can be included and assessed alongside their peers.

Chapter 3, Including Children With Disabilities in Dance Assessment, provides a variety of dance assessments that include children with a variety of disabilities in the cognitive, affective and psychomotor domains.

Chapter 4, Assessing Game Skill Performance, offers different ways to include all students in games so that they can be assessed.

Chapter 5, Establishing Criteria for Assessments, offers a variety of ideas to help teachers develop rubrics so that they can assess all students in a similar way.

Chapter 6, Assessing & Improving Fitness, offers suggestions for assessing students' heart rates, including different methods of heart rate measurement in the classroom setting, and for assessing fitness components through developing personal fitness profiles for students.

Chapter 7, Assessing Aquatics, provides variations of assessment in the aquatic environment.

The book's Appendix contains definitions of categories of students with disabilities referred to within the chapters of the book.

The authors hope that, after reading this book, physical education teachers will be comfortable using the numerous strategies provided to assess all students in the physical education setting.

How to Use This Book

This book is intended to give instructors ideas for modifying assessment so that they meet the physical education needs of all children. To use this book most effectively:

1. Identify the students in your class with unique needs, and use the assessment modifications contained in this book that are appropriate to the skill you're teaching. Implement the UDL approach from the appropriate chapter, as well, to provide various ways to participate in the assessments.

2. Implement the assessment with everyone in your class.

3. Plan your program according to the assessment's outcome for each child.

4. Reassess and determine what improvements and program modifications are needed.

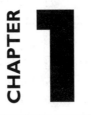

CHAPTER 1

Applying the Universal Design for Learning Approach to Assessment

Lauren J. Lieberman, Ph.D.
The College at Brockport, State University of New York

Assessment is the key to programming and instruction for elementary physical education. Still, physical educators often hesitate to assess student learning (Schiemer, 2000). That might be due to time constraints, lack of personnel or lack of good assessments.

The Importance of Assessment for Everyone

Elementary classroom teachers rely on assessment data for planning curriculum and instruction, and for measuring student progress. Assessments are an important part of the instruction process for all teachers.

Some physical education teachers hesitate to assess because of the vast heterogeneity found in today's classrooms, including children with disabilities who are on individualized education programs (IEPs) or 504 plans, and children with varying backgrounds related to motor skill and experiences. This hesitation is due, frequently, to the lack of assessment tools for children with disabilities and a reluctance to hold students with disabilities accountable for learning. To be sure, assessing such a wide array of students with different skills and needs is difficult. But to teach all children effectively, teachers must ensure that assessment occurs for children with disabilities, even when different assessment approaches or tools are necessary.

Teachers today must devise a variety of ways to assess so that they can determine each child's strengths and areas needing improvement. Only when those assessments are documented can a teacher plan the class and reassess to observe that learning has taken place. But that leads to the question: "How do I assess for the variability of skill in my class?"

What Is the UDL Approach?

One answer to that assessment question is the Universal Design for Learning (UDL) approach. UDL emerged from the architectural design field when federal legislation required universal access to buildings and other structures for people with disabilities. Architects began to design accessibility into buildings and other structures rather than retrofitting standard structures. Curb cuts, for example, enable people in wheelchairs to access the sidewalk while also making travel easier for those using walkers, for parents with strollers, for bicycle riders and for older people who have trouble negotiating curbs (Lieberman, Lytle & Clarq, 2008).

Universal design in learning means that the physical, social and learning environments are designed so that *all* learners are supported in teaching and learning (McGuire, Scott & Shaw, 2006). UDL presents a concept, a set of principles, a framework and a frame of mind that support access for the widest number of people (Odem, Brantlinger, Gersten, Thompson & Harris, 2005). To collect data on each student, the assessment must apply to *all* students. This doesn't mean that each student is assessed the same way, but that the same content is assessed for every child. Teachers can accomplish that in a variety of ways using the UDL approach.

UDL can provide a way to eliminate barriers to learning that students might encounter and can include ramps, bowling ramps, lifts for pools and beepers behind baskets. UDL includes Universally Designed Instruction, such as the use of trained peer tutors, enlarged print or print in Braille, and closed-captioning on videos. The same universal approach can be applied to curriculum (Universally Designed Curriculum) and assessment (Universally Designed Assessment) (Meyer & Rose, 2000; Rose & Meyer, 2002).

How to Incorporate the UDL Approach With Assessments

The three major variables that one must consider before implementing the UDL approach with assessment are the:

1. Attributes of all learners in the class. This might include different ways that some students in the class communicate, including sign language, picture boards or gestures; the way they ambulate, including walkers, crutches, wheelchairs, etc.; or the way they learn, including more time for processing, need for close proximity or the need for repetition.

2. Objectives for the class and for individual students. This can include skill development for a soccer unit, balance and strength for gymnastics, or cooperation for an outdoor adventure class.

3. Modification variables. These include variations to the instruction, rules, equipment or environment when implementing an assessment.

When analyzing learners' attributes, the teacher must consider each child's functional ability and then implement those considerations into the assessment protocol. Modification variables (Lieberman, Lytle & Clarq, 2008) include changing an object's weight, size or type; changing the speed of movement; or changing the skill *(Figure 1.0)*. When instructors plan for assessment, they must consider each learner's attributes before developing or implementing a lesson.

Example: Mrs. Jacobs teaches a 2nd-grade class and is using the Test of Gross Motor Development II (TGMD II) (Ulrich, 2000), a norm-referenced assessment for locomotor and object-control skills. Jamal, who has cerebral palsy and uses a walker, and Brianna, who has a visual impairment, are members of Mrs. Jacob's class. Mrs. Jacobs knows that Jamal can perform every skill in his own way and at his own pace. She knows that Brianna has had some exposure to the skills in the past but needs verbal input and has a preference for red balls with bells inside to help her track the ball.

Mrs. Jacobs employs the UDL approach in her assessment by offering a variety of balls (including red bell balls) for the kicking assessment on the TGMD II, as well as an option to kick from a seated position. She also offers a variety of options on the catching test, including catching a bounce pass, catching from a seated position and catching a beach ball. Mrs. Jacobs also offers a variety of ways to slide, gallop, skip, jump and run. She collects data for every TGMD II test for each child, with help from Brianna's and Jamal's paraeducator and several trained peer tutors.

Keep in mind that, when modifying an assessment that is valid and reliable (such as TGMD II), with the protocol included, the modified test is no longer valid. One can't use the data collected with the existing norms or standards, although one *can* use the results as descriptive data on a child's assessment report and to determine progress. (Assessments in NASPE's Assessment Series have no established validity or reliability and, therefore, can be modified and used with no harm to their validity or reliability.)

Figure 1.0. Examples of the UDL Approach to Assessment

Child's Need	UDL Assessment Approaches
Support in running, due to balance or lack of vision.	• Run along a wall. • Run along a guidewire. • Run with a sighted guide. • Run on a treadmill.
1:1 assessment.	• Train the teacher's aide (paraeducator) (Lieberman, 2007). • Train a peer tutor (3rd grade or above, preferably). • Train parent volunteers on assessment collection techniques.
Variations in speed and direction of the test items.	• Use a bounce pass for catching. • Use a beach ball. • Bat off a tee. • Kick from a sitting position, using a stationary ball. • Skip, using poly spots and verbal cues.
Additional cues in assessment skills, such as object control, balance or locomotor.	• Use visual information, including pictures, demonstrations or posters of a skill or a task-analyzed skill. • Use specific cues to help with specific skill steps, such as "Shoulder to your aid," "Step," "Roll the ball," "Push."

Note: When using any of these approaches, include detailed explanation so that the team knows how the child performed the skill for the assessment.

Using Differentiated Instruction With Assessment

In addition to using the UDL approach, it's important for teachers to use the differentiated instruction concept when assessing. Students comprehend information in various ways, including visually, auditorily, kinesthetically and tactually (Thousand, Villa & Nevin, 2007). Accounting for students' learning styles when assessing allows teachers to collect the most reliable assessments.

Example: Annie needed several demonstrations of each skill performed right in front of her so that she could see and feel the performer. Then, with feedback, she executed the skill. She also needed several practices to understand what she was being asked to do. That was differentiated instruction for her, and she performed to the best of her ability. The assessment was appropriate for her, because she was assessed on the skill and not her *comprehension* of the skill. By taking Annie's attributes into account, her teacher could evaluate Annie's best skills and, therefore, assess what she had learned.

Terms & Techniques

Several terms and techniques are useful when using the UDL approach, including:

1. Modify variables, when necessary. As seen with the previous example, one can modify the equipment, rules and environment to ensure the child's success with the activity. Again, the teacher must consider the child's skills and abilities, which are called "attributes." For example, if a child uses a walker, you might have him complete a half-mile walk instead of a mile run to assess his endurance. Or, you might have him serve a volleyball from half court instead of from the service line, or hit a ball off a tee instead of from a pitch.

As with modifying the circuit for the heart rate monitor assessment in Chapter 6, considering the child's attributes will give the teacher ideas on how to modify variables in the assessment to accommodate the child's needs.

2. Disability awareness. Use this strategy to sensitize other students about disability issues and to ensure that they understand the cause of differences in children with disabilities. Research shows that children without disabilities are more accepting of children with disabilities if they know why those children talk, walk or function differently. Sharing information on a disability's cause, characteristics and function helps peers accept and even embrace the differences that a child with a disability might display. When possible, ask a child with a disability to share that information with the class to the extent that he/she feels comfortable. Then, when you modify the assessment for that child, the others will understand why.

3. Peer tutoring. Different from peer interaction, peer tutoring involves training students — either the same age or older — to assist within the instruction environment (Lieberman & Houston-Wilson, 2009). Whether in an inclusive or a segregated setting, trained peer tutors have been shown to improve skill levels for children with disabilities, as well as helping to increase socialization opportunities. Peer tutors can help with guiding, instruction and feedback, and with giving those children information about the environment. They also can assist with collecting data on simple assessments.

Example: Destiny is in 5th grade, has cerebral palsy and uses a walker. Her teacher trained three peer tutors and included Destiny in the training program. When the teacher assessed swimming, game skills and heart health, the peer tutors helped collect data on Destiny using the rubrics that the teacher gave them. *(See Chapter 5 for more on developing appropriate rubrics.)* They then turned in the scores, which helped the teacher ensure that Destiny was assessed and that she was improving. *(See Lieberman & Houston-Wilson, 2009, for a peer-tutor training program.)*

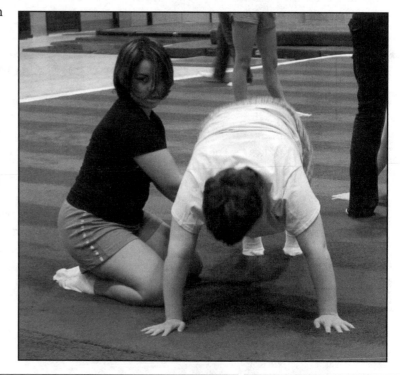

4. Paraeducators. Many children with disabilities have a teacher's aide, also known as a paraprofessional or paraeducator. Paraeducators can perform many of the same functions that peer tutors do in physical education class, including helping with guiding, instructing, offering feedback and giving children with disabilities information about what's happening in the environment. Trained paraeducators also can assist with assessment and data collection.

Example: Patrick was involved in his 4th-grade physical education class. He also happened to have a cognitive disability, as well as a seizure disorder. Mrs. Collier, a paraeducator, assisted in physical education occasionally, but did not assist with instruction or assessment. At the beginning of Patrick's 5th-grade year, the physical education staff conducted a half-day training for the paraeducators. The administration wanted more assessment, and the solution was to have the paraeducators help with data collection.

After the training, Mrs. Collier and the other paraeducators were able to assist with recording data on their students, allowing the teachers to gather more data on the children with and without disabilities. At one station, for example, Mrs. Collier recorded the number of times that Patrick was able to throw a 5-inch ball to hit inside a hula hoop taped on a wall from 10 feet away.

Once Mrs. Collier received the training, Patrick began mastering more skills, and socializing more with his friends, and he knew how much he was learning, most of the time. It also helped his teacher to ensure that the assessments were appropriate and administered as often as necessary. *(See Lieberman, 2007, for a physical education paraeducator training book.)*

5. Physical assistance. The instructor can manipulate a child with a disability through a skill (e.g., tapping the child's knee to prompt him/her to step forward, or moving the child's arm through the front crawl swim motion). Instructors can offer partial physical assistance, as in the two examples above, or total assistance, such as full assistance with a throw or both hands on the child's legs when kicking in a pool. Children with disabilities might need to have their instruction delivered in specific ways for them to understand fully what's being taught or to be assessed with the same instrument as their peers. Teachers who have high expectations for their students must use physical assistance in some instances to elicit the appropriate motor response. It's fine to use physical assistance during an assessment, but teachers must document the amount of assistance applied and where it was delivered for the assessment to be replicated and further learning to be assessed. The hope is that the children eventually will need less physical assistance and do more on their own, when possible.

It's important that the instructor or paraeducator evaluates carefully the skill being taught and what the child can do so that the child isn't offered too much physical assistance.

Example: Hollyn is a 12-year-old girl who has hemiplegic cerebral palsy (paralysis on half of her body) and a visual impairment. When she is in the pool kicking, she often turns on her side due to her hemiplegia. When the instructor physically assists her back and helps her weak leg when kicking, Hollyn can kick for 30 seconds without stopping. Without the assistance, she would turn over and choke on the water. The hopes are that Hollyn works on improving from there and that, the next time she is assessed, she is even more independent.

Summary

Assessment is a cornerstone of instruction. Assessing all children — including those with disabilities, alongside their peers — will allow instructors to determine children's strengths and weaknesses, to plan and to document improvements. Good and appropriate assessments can become part of children's IEPs. With some effort, creativity and support, teachers can assess *all* children.

CHAPTER 2

Assessing Elementary Motor Skills

Lauren J. Lieberman, Ph.D.
The College at Brockport, State University of New York

Renee McCall, M.S. Ed.
North Syracuse Central School District

Assessing motor skills is a basic requirement for any elementary physical education teacher. Motor skills can be assessed in a variety of ways using a variety of different tools. This chapter is designed to help physical educators assess students who might demonstrate clear challenges when attempting to perform skills, and it is intended to complement the assessments suggested in the NASPE Assessment Series book *Assessing Motor Skills in Elementary Physical Education*, by Shirley Ann Holt/Hale (1999).

With a few key tools, physical educators can establish a developmentally appropriate *starting point* for skill development and a successful class experience for all students, including those with disabilities. Strategies for assessing the skill level of students with disabilities will vary greatly based on the child's disability or challenge. This chapter outlines a selection of assessment checklists, along with adaptation and modification guidelines, that teachers can use to establish an appropriate starting point for skill development. It also explores instruction techniques, equipment and communication needs when adapting to the unique cognitive, affective, psychomotor and social needs of students with disabilities.

This chapter employs the UDL approach as discussed in Chapter 1. Using the modifications proposed here will help teachers assess all children on motor skills.

Teacher Observation of Critical Cues: Checklists

In developing an observation checklist, teachers must first identify the critical cues — phrases or individual words that identify and communicate critical features of the skill or task to a child — of the task(s) they are assessing (Rink, 2009). These movement cues help focus children's attention and help them retain the skill.

To provide meaningful instruction, teachers must first recognize that children with various disabilities differ in their learning styles, physical abilities and in the rates at which they process information. Screening children with disabilities is a good place to start in the process of recognizing what they will need. In some instances, teachers will have to modify the cues used to assist children with disabilities, as well as children who have not played or performed the selected skills before.

Cue Modifications

Some children with and without disabilities would benefit from teachers' elaborating on existing or traditional cues. Some examples:

- Include pictures with each cue, along with demonstration. Teachers might need, for example, to show students close-up photos of how to dribble a basketball with the pads of their fingers.

- Use sign language or gestures to deliver the point.

- Allow the child to practice several times before rating him/her on the skill. Some children might take longer than others to associate the cue with the skill. Allow several attempts with the cue and with demonstration before assessing the child.

- Modify checklists according to children's abilities. Instead of giving cues only at the beginning, teachers might need to increase the repetitions and give cues throughout the task to help children process the information. A child who is just learning to dribble, for example, might use the cues "Push, push, catch." Then, the child can progress to "Push, push, push, catch," and so on. That way, the child maintains the ball and uses his/her attention span on three dribbles.

- Offer hand-over-hand assistance, when necessary. That might be the way that the child experiences the skill.

Physical educators might need to add cues for component parts of the skill. In addition to saying "Pads, pads, push, push" in a dribbling drill, for example, the teacher might have to say "Extend" or "Continue."

For further modification, students can perform the dribbling while kneeling, sitting in a chair or on the floor, standing, walking or running. They can use a basketball, a playground ball, Nerf® ball, beach ball or balloon.

Checklist

A checklist — "a statement of the skill and listing of critical cues for a particular grade level and/or class" (Holt/Hale,1999, p. 4) — can prove effective in collecting the information necessary to develop a plan for instruction. An important point: cues to be assessed should not be new to the student; instead, they should be part of the instruction environment from the beginning of the unit.

A checklist of critical cues for the basic dribbling skill could include:

____ "Pads, pads, push, push."

____ "Hand on top."

____ "Waist-high."

____ "Knees bent."

____ "Firm wrists/flexible wrists."

____ "Head up."

Teachers might need to modify the checklists they use for children with disabilities according to each child's abilities. A child with autism and limited attention and control, for example, might need to start out sitting on the floor and dribbling three times with the pads of the fingers. From there, the child can progress to sitting in a chair and dribbling, then standing. At that point, the teacher can include the other component parts in the assessment, such as dribbling the ball at waist height while on one knee. The teacher might need to use that progression to assess children with intellectual disabilities, as well as those with visual impairments. That approach — allowing children to execute skills at various levels — is an example of a UDL approach discussed in Chapter 1, and it will allow each child to start where he/she feels comfortable.

Sample Checklist:

____ Start out in a sitting position and dribble 3-5 times with two hands.

____ In a sitting position, dribble 3-5 times with one hand.

____ In a sitting position, dribble 3 times in a row with the pads of the fingers.

____ Sit in a chair and dribble 3-5 times in a row with the pads of the fingers.

____ Stand and dribble 3-5 times in a row with the pads of the fingers.

You can modify the checklist above for any ability level, adding or removing tasks.

Observation

Observation is an important part of reflective teaching, particularly at the beginning of each class. When observing motor skill performance, the tendency is to see all the things that the student is doing incorrectly. But when assessing motor skills, teachers must remember to focus on observing only one cue at a time and then providing feedback on that single cue. Although *Assessing Motor Skills in Elementary Physical Education* (Holt/Hale, 1999) suggests eight to 10 children per observation group, a smaller group or more observers will help document exactly which part of the checklist each child completed correctly and can help determine what is missing for future instruction. When applying UDL to assessment checklists, teachers might need to ensure that children with disabilities are in a smaller group, or they might need to be observed individually.

Example: A 4th-grade class is being assessed on rolling a ball using the Test of Gross Motor Development II (Ulrich, 2000). The class of 32 children is broken up into groups of eight. The evaluators consist of the teacher, the co-teacher (coming in on her free period), a paraeducator and a parent volunteer. Each evaluator takes one group for this skill *(Figure 2.0).*

Figure 2.0. Sample Checklist for Assessing Frisbee™-Throwing Skills

Child	Skill component	0 or 1
Ariel	1. Grips the Frisbee™ with thumb on top and fingers underneath. 2. Brings arm with Frisbee™ across the chest. 3. Steps forward with throwing-side foot. 4. Follows through and releases the Frisbee™.	_____ _____ _____ _____
Autumn	1. Grips the Frisbee™ with thumb on top and fingers underneath. 2. Brings arm with Frisbee™ across the chest. 3. Steps forward with throwing-side foot. 4. Follows through and releases the Frisbee™.	_____ _____ _____ _____
Gabriel	1. Grips the Frisbee™ with thumb on top and fingers underneath. 2. Brings arm with Frisbee™ across the chest. 3. Steps forward with throwing-side foot. 4. Follows through and releases the Frisbee™.	_____ _____ _____ _____
Justin	1. Grips the Frisbee™ with thumb on top and fingers underneath. 2. Brings arm with Frisbee™ across the chest. 3. Steps forward with throwing-side foot. 4. Follows through and releases the Frisbee™.	_____ _____ _____ _____
Leon	1. Grips the Frisbee™ with thumb on top and fingers underneath. 2. Brings arm with Frisbee™ across the chest. 3. Steps forward with throwing-side foot. 4. Follows through and releases the Frisbee™.	_____ _____ _____ _____
Nadine	1. Grips the Frisbee™ with thumb on top and fingers underneath. 2. Brings arm with Frisbee™ across the chest. 3. Steps forward with throwing-side foot. 4. Follows through and releases the Frisbee™.	_____ _____ _____ _____
Penelope	1. Grips the Frisbee™ with thumb on top and fingers underneath. 2. Brings arm with Frisbee™ across the chest. 3. Steps forward with throwing-side foot. 4. Follows through and releases the Frisbee™.	_____ _____ _____ _____
Steven	1. Grips the Frisbee™ with thumb on top and fingers underneath. 2. Brings arm with Frisbee™ across the chest. 3. Steps forward with throwing-side foot. 4. Follows through and releases the Frisbee™.	_____ _____ _____ _____

Comments: Nadine threw the Frisbee™ from her wheelchair.

Self-Assessment

As described in *Assessing Motor Skills in Elementary Physical Education* (Holt/Hale, 1999), student self-assessments can use the same checklist of critical cues or skill components that the teacher uses during performance observation *(Figure 2.1)*. Students can check off which column next to each component that they think expresses their ability; "I need help with this skill," for example, or "I'm good at this skill" (Holt/Hale, 1999, p.10). For children who are able, having the opportunity to assess their own levels of performance — along with having the opportunity to document their own improvement — is empowering and proves to be a great motivator.

Student self-assessments provide teachers with valuable insight into students' perceptions of their own skill levels; students can rate themselves much lower than their abilities or considerably higher than what the teacher rates them. The peer pressure and subsequent embarrassment that often accompany a group assessment give way to students' ability to identify, record and then set the pace for their own productive and personalized skill development. Using the rubric is an ideal tool for self-assessment, because the skill to be mastered is specific and individualized.

Figure 2.1. Sample Batting Self-Assessment # 1

Instructions: Circle the word that *BEST* describes how often you are able to perform each task.

Description	Evaluation
I can stand at the batting tee with my shoulder facing the target.	Always Sometimes Never
My favorite hand is on top of my other hand on the bat.	Always Sometimes Never
I start with the bat at my shoulder.	Always Sometimes Never
I can swing and step onto my front foot.	Always Sometimes Never
I can follow through with the bat.	Always Sometimes Never

Note, though, that you might need to modify some checklists for children with disabilities for them to be able to self-assess. When applying the UDL approach, keep these points in mind while considering such modifications:

- Using pictures and demonstrations helps determine the success of the target skill. For example, a student with autism might not be able to read or communicate effectively on paper during a self-assessment but can look at a picture next to each skill component and check off "Yes, I do," or "Not yet." *Example:* "My arms are straight when I swing."

- Trained paraeducators can help children determine whether they have mastered the skill and whether they are executing the skill's various components.

- Trained peer tutors can help demonstrate the skills and help children evaluate themselves. For example, using a checklist with pictures, a peer tutor can point and help students focus on the part of the skill performance that they're responding to.

- Using stations with distinct separations will help children know when they're performing different components of a skill. For example, children who can dribble five times in a row at the dribbling station will know that they have "graduated" to the dribbling-while-walking station. Those who can dribble while walking then know that they have "graduated" to the dribbling-while-jogging station.

- Some children might need less information on each checklist, but more checklists. Children who need to know that they are improving, for example, can use one checklist for their "Push, push, catch, push, push, push, catch" until they can dribble five times. Then, they go to the checklist with "Walk five steps while pushing the ball with fingertips."

- Teachers can help children understand better by changing number ratings to smiley faces; thumbs up, sideways or down; or plus and minus signs *(Figure 2.2)*.

Figure 2.2. Sample Batting Self-Assessment # 2

Instructions: Circle the face that *BEST* describes how you feel about how you perform each task.

Description	Evaluation		
I can stand at the batting tee with my shoulder facing the target.	:)	:]	: (
My favorite hand is on top of my other hand on the bat.	:)	:]	: (
I start with the bat at my shoulder.	:)	:]	: (
I can swing and step onto my front foot.	:)	:]	: (
I can follow through with the bat.	:)	:]	: (

Self-Assessment Progressions

In some cases, children can use a progression to evaluate themselves. In that case, they must master the first skill, then move to the next one. That can be a rubric and a checklist of tasks of increasing difficulty or a rating scale.

Below is an example of an individual self-assessment progression designed for a student named Xavier, who has hemiplegic cerebral palsy, as he works to improve his ability to jump rope. This is a good example of using UDL for all students because even children without disabilities sometimes have poor balance and display poor jump-rope skills.

Sample Jump-Rope Self-Assessment Progression # 1

_____ Xavier will step forward over the rope on the floor 5 times while holding on to the wall.

_____ Xavier will jump with both feet over the rope on the floor 5 times while standing next to the wall.

_____ Xavier will leap over the rope on the floor 1 time while standing next to the wall.

_____ With the rope at 6 inches off the floor, Xavier will step forward over it 5 times.

_____ With the rope 6 inches off the floor, Xavier will leap over it 3 times.

_____ Xavier will hold on to the jump rope, swing it over his head and step over it 5 times in a row.

_____ Xavier will hold on to the jump rope, swing it over his head and step over it 10 times in a row.

_____ Xavier will hold on to the jump rope, swing it over his head and jump over it 1 time.

Note: Teachers can modify this checklist to prescribe a certain number of jumps forward and backward, depending upon the student's abilities.

Using rubrics as a form of skill assessment can individualize instruction within a class setting, as each student works on goals specific to his/her needs. Teachers then can facilitate the learning process with instruction cues as each student works on his/her skill task. In Xavier's class, for example, some students were working on jumping rope forward with two feet for 50 jumps (_Sample Jump Rope # 2_); other students were working on jumping one leg at a time for two minutes (the length of a song); and two others were working on a progression similar to Xavier's.

Sample Jump-Rope Self-Assessment Progression # 2

_____ Melissa will jump with both feet over her rope 10 times without stopping.

_____ Melissa will jump with both feet over her rope 30 times without stopping.

_____ Melissa will jump with both feet over her rope 50 times without stopping.

_____ Melissa will jump backward with both feet 10 times without stopping.

_____ Melissa will jump backward with both feet 20 times without stopping.

_____ Melissa will jump backward with both feet 20 times without stopping, then 20 times forward without stopping.

Teachers can apply UDL by using this same rubric in a partner format. Completing the rubric with a partner leads peers to work together to practice and record progress, but also helps students who might have difficulty reading the performance criteria (Lieberman & Houston-Wilson, 2009). *Note:* We suggest that teachers first train peer tutors to ensure appropriate interaction, cues, feedback and expectations.

In this next example, Brooke, who has autism, has a goal of dropping the ball to the floor and picking it up independently as a variation to dribbling. Here is Brooke's self-assessment progression checklist:

_____ 1. Brooke stands independently, holding the ball with two hands.

_____ 2. Brooke drops the ball to the floor.

_____ 3. Brooke picks up the ball, maintaining her balance independently.

_____ 4. Brooke repeats this sequence 3 times.

Student Project/Event Task

Student projects provide an opportunity for teachers to assess students' ability to demonstrate skills in combination and various contexts, as well as their creative application of skill in a dynamic environment (Holt/Hale, 1999). They also lend themselves well to assessing students with disabilities.

Student projects can vary in subject and content, from creating a ball-handling and -dribbling routine in basketball or soccer *(see checklist below)* to a dance or tumbling routine. The basic premise of a project is for the child to make decisions on with whom to work, what skills to include, what rhythm to use, how long the routine will be, what equipment to use, and whether the team should include music.

Children with disabilities can make those decisions themselves — or with help from a teacher or paraeducator — and can be evaluated with their peers on the routine created. Some modifications to consider:

- If the child chooses to perform his/her routine with a peer or two, make sure that they are trained peer tutors or are experienced working with the child.

- Make sure that the child has input into the routine's variables.

- Ensure that the variables are within the child's range of ability.

- Ensure that the assessment used is fair, relative to the child's skill level.

- Determine whether the child needs more practice time.

- Determine whether to use cues, demonstrations and pictures during the routine.

Soccer Checklist Evaluation

P = Present   S = Somewhat   A = Absent

_____ Routine lasted 3-5 minutes.

_____ Routine contained 5 soccer moves learned in class.

_____ Each member of the team participated in the routine.

_____ Clear use of space and levels throughout the routine.

_____ Routine included creativity.

_____ Teamwork was involved in 3 of the 5 previous elements.

Summary of evaluation:

Modification Example: Basketball

Here are some examples of modifications to the example skill of dribbling. Instructors can extend these examples to other skills and assessment situations:

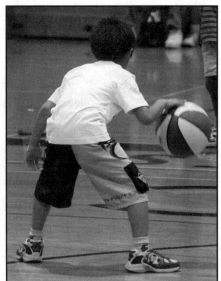

- Suggest that the child embrace the ball against his/her torso with the hands or forearm as it bounces up from the floor each time after a dribble.

- Instruct the child to begin by bouncing a basketball or playground ball against a wall and catching it on the rebound.

- Use a large, light-weight ball with a lot of bounce that a child with cerebral palsy, for instance, can push down on with an open or closed hand or a forearm.

- Attach one clip of a coiled key ring to a punching ball. Attach the other end around the student's wrist. The student can practice the motion of pushing down on the ball repeatedly without feeling the frustration of the ball moving outside of his/her range.

Additional Modifications

Here are some general modifications that teachers can use with a variety of sport skills:

- Substitute a light-weight ball or a playground ball.

- Have the student kneel when first trying to dribble while establishing a more stable base of support.

- Have the student sit in a chair for support, freeing his/her hands for dribbling.

- Use a tray or incline that a child with a severe disability can use to roll a ball toward a target.

- Have the child push up instead of down, by "dribbling" a balloon with a racket or his/her hand(s).

- Use picture cards to help the child visualize the task.

- Use a beeper ball or a ball with a bell in it, for children who are blind or have low vision.

Communication

In many instances, communication is the key to helping children perform a skill to the best of their ability. Communication boards are used commonly to convey necessary motor skills in a sequence for children on the autism spectrum, but they're also helpful for children who have processing or intellectual difficulties. Introducing a communication board or some type of visual direction with pictures will establish a pattern of expected behavior. A communication strip, as it often is called, is a sequence of picture symbols that the instructor can point to as a visual reinforcement to what he/she is asking of the student. In addition, using a sequence of visual symbol(s) provides the structured introduction of tasks to be performed, which often works well for students who need predictability. Here are some symbols to consider:

1. The first symbol can be a picture sign for "Look at me."

2. The second picture can simulate the motion of a person dribbling or bouncing and catching a ball.

3. The third picture can symbolize "Walk," Run" or "Stop," depending on what the teacher wants the student to try next while dribbling.

Teachers can create picture symbols by using computer software programs such as Boardmaker®. If Boardmaker® or a similar program isn't available, creating symbol cards will work just as well. Just laminate simple stick-figure drawings or a photo of another child dribbling a ball.

Summary

Motor skills form the basis for playing sports. All children must learn how to develop a variety of motor skills. With the suggestions from this chapter, teachers can use NASPE's assessment of motor skills for all children.

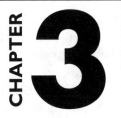

Including Children With Disabilities in Dance Assessment

Ellen M. Kowalski, Ph.D.
Adelphi University

Including dance in the physical education curriculum provides students of all abilities with an opportunity to explore moving in ways that are creative, communicative and expressive. This chapter is intended to complement the assessment ideas presented in the NASPE Assessment Series book *Assessing Dance in Elementary Physical Education* (Cone & Cone, 2005) to teach and assess all children in dance. The chapter addresses the benefits and uses of dance assessments and applies UDL, thereby making assessment appropriate for all students in the class, including students with disabilities.

The chapter reviews the various dance forms (cultural, social and creative); offers a variety of dance assessments for the cognitive, affective and psychomotor domains; and shares a variety of ways to infuse UDL into dance assessment.

In *Assessing Dance in Elementary Physical Education,* Cone and Cone define categories of cultural, social and creative dance forms and align them with the National Standards for Physical Education, as well as including student expectations. The focus of **cultural dance,** the authors state, is that its steps and movements represent the expression of a culture's heritage, traditions, beliefs and values or important events.

The purpose of **social dance,** they write, is to help students learn that "dance is a means to interact positively with others and enjoy moments of sharing as a community." Teaching students to express their personalities through sharing movements common in popular social dance provides a bonding experience and helps students with disabilities learn socially acceptable ways of interacting with others in an inclusive setting.

Cone and Cone define **creative dance** as new and original dances developed by students, teachers or both. Children can explore and organize movements about varied topics, including emotions, stories, animals, holidays, seasons, monsters, etc.

As the following section explains, within each of those dance forms lies a variety of dance assessments for the cognitive, affective and psychomotor domains.

Assessment: Who, What & When

Many children with disabilities display developmental delays in body and spatial awareness, auditory and visual processing and memory, coordination and self-esteem, and they have difficulty with self-expression and communication. Because children with disabilities display those difficulties, it's important to first identify *basic abilities* required in dance as part of the assessment process (Kaufmann, 2006). Understanding a student's basic dance abilities can help teachers select the appropriate assessment instrument and modify it so that it accommodates each individual student's needs.

In *Inclusive Creative Movement and Dance* (2006), Karen Kaufmann presents five basic ability categories that physical educators should assess:

1. Body awareness.

2. Spatial awareness.

3. Listening (movement cues and music).

4. Watching (movement cues).

5. Visualization skills and recall.

Body awareness relates to children's internal map of their body parts and their relationship to one another. That awareness is critical in developing an internal sense of alignment, or how to position one's body without the use of vision. *Example:* knowing, without looking, that you are standing with your feet parallel, shoulder-width apart and knees bent.

Spatial awareness relates to children's awareness of personal space and their relationship to others.

Listening involves being able to respond to tempos, accents and phrasing of music, as well as to teachers' instructions.

Watching involves being able to see and imitate the teacher's demonstration.

Visualization skills and recall refer to the ability to use imagery to translate cognitive information into movement. In her book, Kaufmann also provides a four-point rubric *(Figure 3.0)* that teachers can use to assess students' abilities in each of the five dance ability categories.

Figure 3.0. Sample Rubric for Assessing Spatial Awareness

Basic	Developing	Emerging	Accomplished
Minimal awareness of the body's personal and group space. Child is challenged to move independently.	Has basic awareness of personal and group space. Moves independently through space but needs extra time to perform task.	Has a developing awareness of personal and group space. Moves through space using a variety of movements. Able to demonstrate pathway, direction and level changes but needs clarification.	Able to move through space using a variety of movements in a variety of pathway, direction and level changes; moves in a coordinated and intentional manner.

— Adapted, with permission, from K. Kaufmann, 2006, p. 19, *Inclusive Creative Movement and Dance,* Human Kinetics.

Including Children With Disabilities in Dance Assessment

As discussed in Chapter 1, using UDL ensures that the teacher knows the attributes of all children in the class. That knowledge will help the teacher offer variables in assessments that all children can use. Only when all attributes are addressed will all children be able to participate and be assessed.

The assessment tools presented in NASPE's *Assessing Dance in Elementary Physical Education* (Cone & Cone, 2005) are inclusive for all children, from low-skilled to moderately skilled movers. The following section explores why the assessments are inclusive, and it provides additional suggestions for modifying them to include students with disabilities.

In the book, Cone and Cone make three important suggestions:

1. *Everyone* in the class should be involved in dance assessment.

2. Dance assessment should target not only the psychomotor domain or physical performance; it should assess all domains.

3. Dance assessment should employ a variety of assessment formats.

Involving Everyone in Dance Assessment

Cone and Cone offer a variety ways to involve *all learners* in the class in dance assessment, including teachers, peers and students using self-assessment. Involving students in creating assessments, assessing one another and assessing oneself aids and supports an inclusive environment. Putting together a dance assessment with the teacher and other children helps create a sense of ownership that's important to developing self-esteem. Involving children in assessing one another not only helps them work on communication skills, it also facilitates social interaction.

Assessing All Domains

Although determining children's ability to perform steps and movement is the focus of dance assessment, the psychomotor domain should not be the only domain used. Unlike assessment of individual and fundamental skills, dance uses expression in all three domains — cognitive, affective and psychomotor — and is important to applying the UDL concept to assessing all children. Assessing children's ability to perform individual movements or a dance sequence allows teachers to determine improvement in coordination, balance, strength, perceptual ability, etc., but it also requires cognitive understanding and memory.

Children have different levels of ability and, although they might not be able to demonstrate a dance well, they can be assessed on other aspects of the dance. A student with severe difficulty in balance or coordination might be able to demonstrate understanding of the dance through written and verbal expression, such as describing the steps in the correct sequence or writing about the history or culture the dance conveys. Students also can demonstrate comprehension within the affective domain by interpreting emotions expressed in a dance or creating a dance for their peers to perform.

Employing a variety of methods for assessing dance knowledge and ability is essential to applying UDL. Using multiple assessment formats not only provides teachers the opportunity to assess holistically but also provides the flexibility to easily accommodate students of varying ability levels, including students with disabilities.

The following section explores selected assessment instruments that Cone and Cone recommend for dance, with suggestions for applying UDL and making them more inclusive for students with disabilities.

Checklists

Teachers can use checklists for teacher, peer or self-assessment with ease, since they require a simple "Yes" or "No" response to each item. And checklists can record students' ability to perform dance steps, such as an allemande in square dance, or an entire dance, such as the troika.

When using checklists for peer or student self-assessment, teachers should, whenever practical, apply UDL by including a picture representation in addition to the word(s). Adding pictures to words creates a visual representation and helps make the words more concrete for children who are non-verbal or for those with processing deficits. If some students have difficulty reading the questions, have all students complete the checklist with a partner.

Journal Writing

Journal writing is effective for assessing the cognitive and affective domains by having children write or draw responses to questions. Teachers should use this format for children with disabilities who are unable to perform the movements well. Use peer tutors to assist students who might be able to verbalize but are unable to write, or for children who have difficulty reading the questions.

Tests & Quizzes

When applying UDL to assessing cognitive learning and/or positive dispositions, teachers should use tests for all children, especially for those with physical disabilities who are unable to perform certain movements. A child with a physical disability, for example, might not be able to perform certain dance steps but can demonstrate knowledge about the dance or emotions expressed in the dance through a written test *(Figure 3.1)*.

Note that checklists and journal writing, as well as tests or quizzes requiring written expression, might not be appropriate for children with processing deficits, autism or cognitive disabilities. This doesn't mean that teachers shouldn't use tests and quizzes to assess children's cognitive ability; only that they might need to modify them to use verbal description or non-verbal expression, such as pictures. Use peer tutors to assist

---

Figure 3.1. Teacher Assessment in the Cognitive and Affective Domains: Quiz on Facts and Feelings About Square Dance

Square Dance Test • Grade 4 • Directions: Circle your answer.

Name: _____

1. A regular square dance formation is composed of how many dancers?   4   8   12   10

2. The partners with their backs to the music are known as couple number: 1   2   3   4

3. Square dance originated in the United States.   True   False

4. With a partner, list three square dance movements that you learned in class.

1. _____   2. _____   3. _____

5. My favorite dance is _____.

— Adapted from *Assessing Dance in Elementary Physical Education*, Cone & Cone (2005), National Association for Sport and Physical Education.

students with cerebral palsy who can vocalize but are unable to write. For children who have difficulty reading the questions or for those with autism who do not speak, insert diagrams and color-coded responses for clarification, wherever possible.

Webs, Maps & Diagrams

This format is an example of UDL, and teachers can use it to assess children who are not able to perform the required movements. Teachers should use **webs** when assessing the cognitive and/or affective domain for children with physical disabilities who are unable to perform the movements or students who are non-verbal and are unable to express the appropriate response. *Example:* Ask students to fill in a blank concept web identifying the various ways to perform a turn *(Figure 3.2)*.

When assessing a child with autism who has difficulty communicating vocally, teachers can use the same web a little differently. The student can watch a peer perform a creative dance. Then, using a completed dance web, the teacher can ask the student to show the ways that the peer performed the dance movement, while pointing out the appropriate movement words. Also, teachers might find it beneficial to color-code a web's movement words for students who have difficulties with memory or visual processing during instruction. Color-coding allows students to associate each color word with an individual movement. Then, using the same color-coded words during assessment helps students remember the movement word and still permits the teacher to see whether the student demonstrates comprehension.

Teachers also can assess children's comprehension of dance concepts by having them draw **maps** of their dance. For example, a child with cerebral palsy can use a map to show the pathways and movements used in his/her creative dance *(Figure 3.3)*.

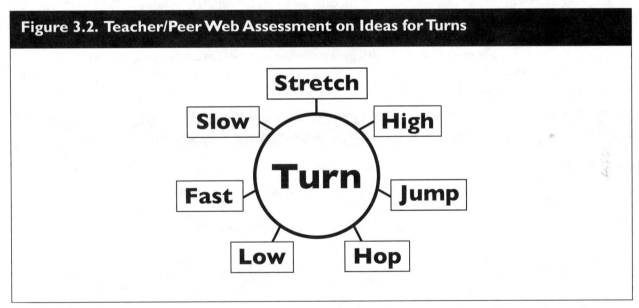

Figure 3.2. Teacher/Peer Web Assessment on Ideas for Turns

— Adapted from *Assessing Dance in Elementary Physical Education,* Cone & Cone (2005), National Association for Sport and Physical Education.

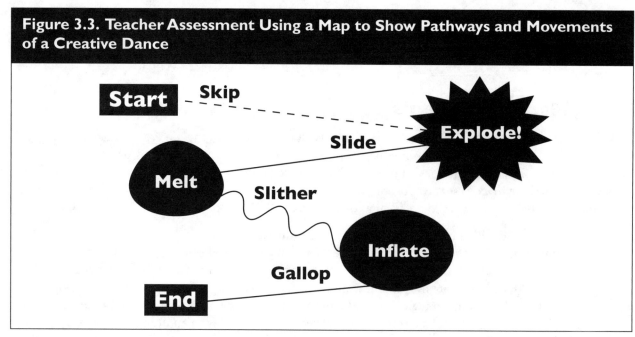

Figure 3.3. Teacher Assessment Using a Map to Show Pathways and Movements of a Creative Dance

— Adapted from *Assessing Dance in Elementary Physical Education,* Cone & Cone (2005), National Association for Sport and Physical Education.

Rating Scales

Teachers can use rating scales as a teacher, peer or self-assessment in all three domains. Peers also can read questions to their partners as they complete an assessment of each other. Adding pictures or symbols, whenever practical, to enhance the meaning of each rating helps make the rating more concrete, especially for children who are non-verbal and those with processing deficits. For example, a student with Down syndrome might not be able to read or communicate effectively on paper during a self-assessment but can demonstrate thoughts and feelings by using a rating scale with symbols *(Figure 3.4).*

Figure 3.4. Student Self-Assessment Checklist in the Psychomotor Domain

Name: _____

Place an "X" in the box that describes your performance in the Balloon Dance.

Held beginning shape for a count of three (3).	I did really well ⊞	I need more practice ⊟
Moved smoothly from small to big.	I did really well ⊞	I need more practice ⊟
Used two different locomotor movements.	I did really well ⊞	I need more practice ⊟
Changed level using good body control.	I did really well ⊞	I need more practice ⊟
Held end shape for a count of three (3).	I did really well ⊞	I need more practice ⊟

— Adapted from *Assessing Dance in Elementary Physical Education,* Cone & Cone (2005), National Association for Sport and Physical Education.

Exit Slips

Teachers can use exit slips at the end of class to assess the cognitive domain (Graham, Holt/Hale & Parker, 2004). The teacher asks students to write the answer to a question about the dance or lesson on a 3 x 5 card. *Example:* "Name or draw one color and one shape that you used in your dance." Providing the option of drawing is a UDL approach that teachers should use when the class includes students who are non-verbal or have communication/speech difficulties.

Teach-Backs

This format assesses students' ability to teach a dance or part of a dance to their peers (Steffen & Grosse, 2003). Teachers should use this to assess cognitive and affective domains, especially for students with physical disabilities who are unable to perform the movements. A student with spina bifida, for example, can demonstrate knowledge of the dance as he/she instructs a peer in performing the dance steps and pathways.

Drawing

Having students create a visual image to express their experience of the lesson is another way to assess their understanding of the dance. Using drawing can be effective in assessing cognitive and affective domains, especially for students with autism and communication disorders who are unable to express themselves well using words. A student with intellectual disabilities might not be able to remember or perform an entire dance sequence but can identify the emotions communicated through the dance by drawing a picture.

Modifications for Including Children With Disabilities in Dance

To ensure that they can assess all children in the class fairly, teachers should apply UDL by first making the dance instruction accessible to all children in the class. As discussed in Chapter 1, when applying UDL, the teacher first determines the attributes of every child in the class. That knowledge will help in offering variations within assessments for all children.

It's important to make certain that any modification used during instruction also is applied during the assessment process. The following list of general modifications and modifications by disability category provides ideas for including children with disabilities both during instruction *and* assessment (Boswell, 2005; Lieberman & Houston Wilson, 2003; Kaufmann, 2006; Kowalski, 2000).

General Modifications

1. Children with different kinds of disabilities — physical, learning, behavior and cognitive — might process information more slowly. (This also applies for ESL children and for students who are not well coordinated.) Allow for extra time to process and repeat instructions before practice or assessment.

2. Because all children — including those with disabilities — have different modality preferences or might have disrupted sensory feedback, teachers should give verbal, visual, tactile and kinesthetic cues to support understanding instructions and performance prior to assessment.

3. Trained peers, cross-age tutors or paraeducators can support students physically through the dance movement. When assessing the cognitive and not the psychomotor domain (e.g., memory of a dance sequence), the purpose of the peer or paraeducator is not to prompt the child but to support him/her as he/she performs the dance.

4. Slow the pace of the dance. Performing the dance a slower pace — both during instruction and assessment — reduces the motor and processing demand.

5. When assessing ability to perform dance steps and not the dance sequence, add visual cues such as poly spots, arrows or colored pinnies to identify spatial orientation or paths.

6. Provide a variety of supports, such as a wall, railing, chair, stool, etc., for any student who has difficulty stepping and/or balancing in place.

Modifications for Children With Physical Disabilities

1. Match children with physical disabilities with a trained peer or cross-age tutor to physically support each child through the dance movement (Lieberman & Houston-Wilson, 2009). A peer tutor, for example, can maintain contact with the child as he/she responds to calls during a square dance assessment. Using a peer can provide a natural way to include a student in the dance assessment who might require help to stand or to undertake a movement.

    Note: For dances performed individually, such as line dances, the teacher can put the entire class in pairs for the dance so that the child with the peer tutor doesn't stand out.

2. Replace movements that a child can't perform while keeping the same count. During a line dance, for example, a student using a wheelchair can bend his/her body to the left and back to substitute for stepping out to the left and back; or if the child can't turn all the way around, he/she can step right, left and right in place in the same amount of time. That way, the child is moving continuously while his/her peers move around, and the teacher can assess rhythm ability to stay on the count. Students using wheelchairs can lift their arms over their heads explosively to substitute for a jump.

3. Modify or eliminate sections of a dance that a child cannot perform and assess him/her on an abbreviated version using movements that he/she *can* perform. For example, a student using a wheelchair can't lie on his/her front to perform a bear walk but can push his/her wheelchair with two feet at the same time as the others are performing the bear walk.

4. Provide support options (wheelchairs, walkers, chairs, stools, etc.) for children who are ambulatory but have balance or mobility issues. A student with cerebral palsy who has lower-leg braces and walks with a scissor gait, for example, can rest his/her hand on the back of a chair for support when performing an aerobic routine.

5. Use tactile and kinesthetic cues or physical assistance to support understanding during instruction (psychomotor domain). Because children with physical disabilities often have disrupted sensory feedback from their bodies (Kelly, 2011; Sugden & Keogh, 1990), a tactile or physical prompt is more effective than a verbal cue. Some students might need physical assistance to understand the skill or to be able to perform at all. Lightly touching or lifting a child's elbow, for example, can help him/her remember to push his/her arms diagonally back and lunge, allowing the teacher to assess performance of the movement.

Modifications for Children With Cognitive & Learning Disabilities

1. When assessing the psychomotor domain, teachers should vocalize and give cues for moving particular body parts or areas of the body. *Example:* Jason has an intellectual disability; he needs short, concise cues. When Jason is to perform a marching motion, the cue is "March." When he is to touch his elbow with the opposite knee, the cue is "Elbows." Short cues like that for a specific count —

four or eight, for example — can help the child remember the dance movements. It will help, also, if the all parts of the dance are cued and performed in the same order. If the dance involves "March," then "Elbows," then "Airplane motion," it should follow the same order each time. Using short cues and keeping the order consistent can ensure that the child is assessed on performance and rhythm, rather than memory.

2. Keep the dance step sequences short to help reduce the processing demand and to allow assessment of performance and rhythmic ability.

3. For children who display poor body awareness, tie a bright scarf around body parts to help with which limb to use in performing movement concepts. One child might have a red scarf on his right hand, for example, and a blue one on the left. The instructor can say "Circle the arm with the red scarf," or "Wave the arm with the blue scarf," etc., to assess the child's ability to perform the dance movement but minimize reliance on right/left concepts.

4. Use pictures of body parts, areas of the body and specific actions/movements to support spoken/written instructions or responses.

5. Use physical prompts or touch (tactile) with spoken cues.

6. Reduce reliance on verbal instructions by providing diagrams, signs or videos to demonstrate the dance that the child is to perform.

7. Limit the amount of reading material.

8. For students with attention deficit disorder (ADD), flashing the lights or a flashlight can help draw and refocus their attention when necessary, allowing the teacher to assess dance performance.

9. Manipulate the student's body part to support visual demonstration. *Example:* Suki has learning disabilities. Often, she learns skills easier with a visual cue and then the instructor moves her body in that motion to reinforce what she learned. Suki's peer tutor taught her a side-slide to the right. She demonstrated it, then moved her legs through the motion slowly to reinforce the motion. Suki understood what was asked and performed the movement faster and faster so that, when assessed, she was able to perform the dance steps as part of the group with her peer tutor providing only visual cues.

Modifications for Children With Autism Spectrum Disorders

1. Use picture cues to help identify movements and/or sequence of dance (psychomotor domain), allowing assessment of the physical movement but reducing the reliance on vocal cueing. Remember that students on the autism spectrum often are poor auditory learners and process information primarily visually, and that they might have difficulty with transitions or change. For all of those reasons, as well as for others, it's helpful to add pictures as much as possible to assessments *(Figure 3.5)*.

Figure 3.5. Providing Pictures to Show Movements Expected to Be Performed in Teacher-Assessment Checklist

Name: _____

Can you make your body move like each of the items below?

1. Airplane   2. Bunny   3. Race Car

4. Butterfly   5. Balloon   6. Snake

7. Ball   8. Elephant

— Adapted from *Assessing Dance in Elementary School,* Cone & Cone (2005), National Association for Sport and Physical Education.

2. Use pictures of a body part, an area of the body and specific actions/movements to show dance movements that the child is expected to perform (psychomotor domain).

3. Identify the child's preferences for type of music, tempo and rhythmic pattern, and use them as part of creating a dance and dance assessment. For example, build in a student's rocking and flapping hands in a rhythmic pattern as a part of a dance, which allows the teacher to assess the cognitive and psychomotor domains.

4. Use tactile and kinesthetic cues to support student understanding of instructions and performance (psychomotor domain).

5. Allow for extra processing time (psychomotor, cognitive and affective domains). Sometimes, a child will need several seconds to process what he/she is being asked to perform. Slow the dance's pace to reduce the processing demand yet allow the child to demonstrate the movements (psychomotor domain) being assessed. *Example:* Slowing an eight-count song to a four-count song with half the number of the beats.

6. If a child is hypersensitive to sound, lower the music volume or allow the child to perform the dance without music.

7. Use poly spots and arrows to assist the child in where to stand and/or identify spatial orientation or direction of travel.

8. In partner dances, use colored pinnies to help students identify their partners.

9. Use a trained peer tutor or paraeducator to help keep students on task.

Modifications for Children With Sensory Impairments

Blind & Visually Impaired Students

Remember that many students who are legally blind have some residual vision. Find out what they can see and make use of whatever vision they do have by using larger objects/print, and neon or bright colors.

1. Ensure visual contact. Make sure that the teacher or peer who is demonstrating knows exactly how far to stand from the child so he/she can see. Children who are visually impaired might need a peer to stand very close with a specific-color shirt to help them maintain a specified distance with a partner or classmate during the dance assessment.

2. Reduce glare from windows and lights during instruction and assessment to maximize available vision.

3. Reduce ambient/distracting noise, when possible, to help children hear the dance instructions.

4. Pair students who are visually impaired with peers who can describe the steps/movement, or read the test question or task to be assessed (cognitive, affective and psychomotor domains).

5. Use tactile and kinesthetic cues to support understanding verbal instructions and performance (psychomotor domain). When teaching the dance, for example, the instructor manipulates the student's body part in that motion to provide a kinesthetic cue to reinforce the verbal instructions. During assessment, provide only tactile cues (light touch) to support instructions for performance. If more support is necessary, document it in the assessment (Lieberman, 2011).

Deaf & Hard-of-Hearing Students

Remember that many students who are deaf have some residual hearing. Find out how much they can hear and make use of whatever hearing they do have by using drums, speakers, etc., and gain visual attention using lights and neon or bright colors.

1. Flash the lights to signal the start/stop of a dance or to draw and refocus the child's attention.

2. During instruction and assessment, clap to the beat so that the child can see the timing and cadence of the dance steps that he/she is to perform.

3. Provide amplification for the student, if appropriate. During instruction and assessment, place speakers on a wooden floor to enhance vibration.

4. Have the child hold a balloon to feel the beat of the music to which he/she is performing through the vibrations in the balloon.

5. Reduce ambient noise to maximize the student's available hearing.

Summary

Many children with various disabilities display developmental delays in self-esteem, body and spatial awareness and coordination, and they have difficulty expressing themselves and communicating. Using UDL to assess dance activities ensures that all students can have the opportunity to explore skills and abilities, enhance self-esteem and promote social interaction, and develop spatial awareness and coordination in ways that are creative and expressive (Kowalski, 2000).

By applying simple modifications to a variety of assessment formats and assessing dance ability in all domains, teachers can include students with disabilities in dance instruction and in dance assessment.

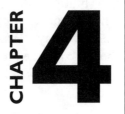

Assessing Game Skill Performance

Lauren J. Lieberman, Ph.D.
The College at Brockport, State University of New York

The purpose of teaching games is to ensure that children have the skills and knowledge to participate successfully in sports and activities throughout their lifetimes. When faced with a student or students with disabilities, elementary school physical education teachers need to make modifications to games so that *all* students can use their functional skills to participate.

This chapter is intended to complement the NASPE Assessment Series book *Games Stages and Assessment* (2007), by David E. Belka, and to present ways to teach and assess game skills for elementary school children, including students with disabilities. Teachers will gain valuable insight on how to assess every child in the class — including those with special needs — on the games taught throughout the school year.

This chapter:

- Reviews the assessments prescribed in *Games Stages and Assessment* and the variety of ways they are used.

- Explores the first three stages of the assessments in *Games Stages and Assessments*.

- Shares a variety of ways to infuse the UDL approach into using the games stages assessments.

- Provides a variety of examples for modifying those assessments.

The ideas presented in NASPE's *Games Stages and Assessment* outline how to assess different levels of sport skills in a logical and sequential order *(Figure 4.0)*. The first two levels of game stages comprise the first component of assessing sport.

Stage 1 focuses on assessing children's performance of individual skills.

Stage 2 focuses on assessing children's performance of a series of skills with competency and thought.

In the second component, **Stages 3 & 4** focus on using the skills to execute tactics in competitive situations. That includes psychomotor skills, cognitive abilities and affective components. The appropriateness of these games stages and assessing them is that they can facilitate the transition from skill learning and cooperative play to beginning competitive play. Because Stage 4, typically, is used with older players, we will not discuss it in depth, as this book is designed for teaching and assessing elementary-age children.

Figure 4.0. The Content of Each Stage		
Stage 1	**Stage 2**	**Stage 3**
Psychomotor Cognitive	Psychomotor Cognitive	Psychomotor Cognitive Affective

This chapter will employ the UDL approach discussed in Chapter 1 as the basis for inclusion. What follow are general modifications that teachers can use throughout assessing games stages.

General Modifications for Assessing Games Stages

1. Use peer tutors and/or paraeducators for instruction, feedback and assessment for some children. This additional instruction and feedback will aid the learning process and will help in assessing children with additional needs. *Note:* Paraeducators also can help students with their sportsmanship and team support, as well as with cognitive testing.

2. Use modifications (e.g., ball size, texture, weight and sound), when necessary. *Example:* Stuart has cerebral palsy and has limited movement in his legs and arms. The teacher took some air out of the soccer ball for the soccer unit. (The teacher also could put 6 oz. of sand in the ball to slow it down.) Stuart's Stage 1 of skill development was easy, because the ball didn't move far when he kicked it and he could dribble under control around cones. Stuart was able to practice combining dribbling and shooting (Stage 2) and played in small-sided games, including 3 v 3, with the underinflated ball. That modification gave him many opportunities to work on his game skills in a game situation (Stage 3).

3. Use physical assistance, if necessary, to help children perform certain skills such as holding a bat, gripping a ball or volleying a ball. Some children will need the assistance to understand how to perform certain skills, and others will be able to participate only with assistance. Teachers should document, on the assessment, the amount of physical support given and where it was given. *Example:* Suki is in grade 4, has low vision and has had limited time playing volleyball. During instruction, her physical education teacher taught her by moving her through the motions of a serve, a bump and a set. For the purposes of learning the skills, she was taught with physical assistance. For the game, Suki was allowed to serve the volleyball with bells, and a peer caught the ball for her and guided her to the net, and she was permitted to throw the ball over the net. Because physical assistance was used to teach the skills and for guidance, those elements must be a part of the assessment.

   Some children who have cerebral palsy, an intellectual disability or paralysis can benefit from physical assistance for activities. This is necessary and preferred to exclusion, and must be documented for assessment purposes. Documentation also is necessary for legal purposes. For example, if a child says that a teacher touched her and you show that she learns and participates with physical assistance, documentation will ensure that you can answer questions from parents or administrators.

4. Add physical education classes, when necessary, to help children with disabilities learn the skills offered in the units. *Example:* Brianna, who has spina bifida and uses a walker, is in grade 6, and her class is about to learn badminton for the first time. Brianna now takes an additional physical education class every week so that she can learn the court, the racquet, the birdie, the rules and the game tactics. Thus, when her class is taught how to serve, she already knows how far she has to stand from the net, and the form and strategy involved while performing from her walker. Instead of coming to physical education class already behind her peers in trying to understand the game's concepts and her abilities, Brianna works on the same skills that the rest of the class is working on.

The assessment of games stages lends itself well to children of all abilities for many reasons. In Stage 1, the focus is on learning, improving and practicing the single skills of receiving, sending and controlling objects. Examples can include throwing, catching, striking and kicking. In the next section, we list some advantages of using game play assessments, which should make clear the appropriateness of diverse classes and classes of children with disabilities, particularly for Stage 1.

Advantages of Using Stage 1 of Games Stages Assessments in All Elementary-Level Physical Education Classes

1. The assessment of skills is developmental and begins with an easy task, such as catching a high-arcing ball, and moves on to more complex tasks, such as catching a low-arcing ball from farther away. This progression works well for children with disabilities, because they usually can perform the task within their own ability levels (e.g., throwing with a scoop, throwing a ball in a sock) and can challenge themselves (e.g., catching from farther away; catching a higher- or faster-thrown ball; throwing through a hula hoop, then throwing into a 12-inch ring) at their own pace.

2. The skills are listed *(Figures 4.1 and 4.2)* and presented as a task analysis, and children are given a score for each level that they reach. The score provides a concrete reference from which children can see their progress and helps provide motivation to work toward the next level. The score is a way of reinforcing learning and achieving basic elements of skills. Teachers can create this type of task analysis for any skill that needs to be assessed.

   Teachers can apply this type of task analysis to any skill, from easy ones such as a throw to ones as complex as a volleyball spike. What's most important is documenting what the child can do and what variations he/she might use, such as from a sitting position, distance from the net or base, and any variations in equipment used. Teachers can write that in the comments section.

3. We recommend that teachers conduct some of the assessments with pictures. Pictures lend themselves well to all learning, but are especially beneficial for students with intellectual/cognitive disabilities and the autism spectrum.

Figure 4.1. Sample Task Analysis for Throwing a Tennis Ball

Name: Jose is a 7-year-old student with cerebral palsy. Jose was given three trials to ensure that he exhibited each of the skills designated below.	From: **X** Sitting __ Standing	Ball type: __ Tennis __ Bean bag **X** Yarn ball	Comments:
Does the child:	**Yes (1)**	**No(0)**	
Move the body with body rotation?	1		Moves stiffly with blocked rotation, yet does rotate.
Hold the ball mainly in the palm of the hand?	1		
Show evidence of weight transfer on the legs?	0		Shows poor balance.
Throw by stepping with the foot opposite the hand?	0		Throws with wide stance, unable to take a step.
Follow through?	1		
Total out of 5	3 of 5 = 60 percent		**Note:** Can score with or without including total percentage of success.

Figure 4.2. Sample Task Analysis for Kicking a Soccer Ball

Name: Miriam is a 6-year-old with autism. She was given three trials to show that she can perform at the following skill level.	From: __ Sitting **X** Standing	Ball type: __ Soccer __ Playground **X** XLarge Therapy	Comments:
Does the child:	**Yes (1)**	**No(0)**	
Move using a three-step approach?	0		Uses two steps.
Plant foot next to the ball?	1		
Shift weight forward?	1		Kicks standing straight up, yet does shift weight.
Kick with the instep of the foot?	1		
Follow through?	1		Trouble with balance.
Total out of 5	4 of 5 = 80%		Note: Can score with or without including total percentage of success.

4. Most assessments like the ones in Figures 4.1 and 4.2 should include a comments section, and teachers can add information about the performance by children with disabilities. As in Figure 4.1, for example, the teacher can add comments to help put a child's difficulty with certain skills into context.

5. The lead teacher doesn't always have the time or the ability to assess all students in the class. But peers, paraeducators and students themselves can conduct the assessments. Assessments like the samples above are clear, discrete and measurable and can be conducted easily by people other than the lead teacher. Peer and self-assessments are for feedback (formative). Only trained teachers should conduct summative assessments.

6. Cognitive pieces are tied into each skill, and students need to think about and answer questions about their own skill execution. That helps guide children to focus on and process feedback from their own bodies.

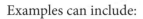

Examples can include:

- What do you have to do to make the ball go the farthest? How do you have to kick to do that?

- Does a heavy ball or a light ball move faster?

- Should you keep your legs straight or bent when kicking?

- Is it easier to kick to a teammate who is running or walking?

- Explain why you selected your answer.

Sample Modifications for Stage 1

- Execute the skill from a standing or sitting position.

- Use balls of different size, weight, color and texture, relevant to the student's abilities.

- Deflated balls will roll slower, lessening the need for movement.

- Add sand to inflated balls to slow their movement.

- Use different-size long-handled implements related to student needs. If a student cannot grip at all, he/she can use the hand only to hit the ball from a tee or from a pitch, or the teacher can use a Velcro® strap to attach the implement to the student's hand.

- Use a ball on a string so that the student doesn't have to run after it. Tie the string to his/her wrist or his/her wheelchair.

Stage 2 of games stages assessment deals more with combinations of skills (e.g., dribbling to shooting) and decisions about which skills to use (e.g., whether to hit a forehand or a backhand in tennis, and a forearm or overhead pass in volleyball). *Note:* This level of decision-making might be best for grade 3 and above.

Transitioning from learning one skill to choosing between skills or linking from one skill to another is not easy. The sample assessment for Stage 2 *(Figure 4.3)* has a very clear practice assessment that uses a Likert scale to determine how well each child is able to accommodate the two skills and/or determine which skill to use (Belka, 2007). It even includes a place to comment on what might help the learner acquire the skills. This assessment is easy to use with children with disabilities.

For the dribbling-to-shooting combination of skills, teachers can apply the UDL approach in the following way. Intersperse 10 cones over 30 feet, with three different-size baskets (one trash can with a backboard and basket attached, a modified basket at a height of eight feet with a wide rim, and a 10-foot regulation basket). Children can perform the combination of dribbling and shooting from an advanced level of dribbling at high speed through the cones and shooting at the 10-foot basket, to dribbling with two hands through cones and shooting at the eight-foot basket, to pushing a student's chair the length of the cones and having the child shoot at the shoulder-level garbage can basket.

The student can choose the complexity, but the assessment should measure or target the smoothness of the combination of dribble to shot.

In tennis, one Stage 2 combination/decision skill would be changing from a forehand to a backhand. Teachers can employ the UDL approach by varying the distance and the type of equipment (e.g., a regulation-size tennis ball, a large foam tennis ball or a balloon). The assessment can still measure students' ability to combine the skills smoothly, but, by modifying the equipment and distance, teachers can include all students in the assessment.

Teachers can make the modifications before class, during the practice, if needed, or after the initial practice to ensure that each child is challenged, yet successful.

Examples of Modifications to Stage 2 Assessments:

- Slow the game's pace by deflating the ball, using a ball that moves slower (e.g., a beach ball) or slowing other students by using carpet squares or tying knees together (i.e., simulating cerebral palsy).

- Vary the distance to the target (e.g., a closer free throw, a shorter distance between bases, or serving closer to the net in volleyball, badminton or tennis).

- Add a support person (e.g., paraeducator or peer tutor) to help children make game decisions, perhaps with cues, such as forehand, forehand, backhand, etc.

- Show short videos of when to make certain game decisions (e.g., whether to shoot, dribble or pass the ball in basketball; when to bump in volleyball; or how close to the hockey goal one should be to shoot).

- Add visual cues (e.g., cones or poly spots) at any time to show children from where to shoot in hockey or basketball.

Figure 4.3. Sample Stage 2 Early Practice Assessment for Soccer Trap & Pass

Performer's Name: _____ Observer: _____

Date: _____ Combination of skills: _____

Rating scale: Circle the most appropriate number beside each statement:

1 = Can be seen in almost all or 100 percent of tries; very consistent.

2 = Evident in 80 percent or most of tries; consistent.

3 = Evident in about 40 percent to 60 percent of tries; variable, not consistent.

4 = Evident in 10 percent to 30 percent of the tries; inconsistent, usually not planned.

5 = Not evident.

Check 1

____   In a drill (slow-motion)

____   In a small-sided game

____   In a scrimmage

____   Other:

Document the date that student accomplishes each skill	**Date**
Trap & pass from a slow-moving ball toward stationary player.	_____
Trap & pass from an average-moving ball toward stationary player.	_____
Trap & pass from fast-moving ball toward running player.	_____
Trap & pass a ball moving away from body to a running player.	_____
Trap & pass a ball at top speed to player running away.	_____

Describe any extraneous movements observed. How can they be reduced?
Use strapping (wide ace bandages or belts) to stabilize, if needed.

Provide one idea to help the student transition between the two skills.

Comments:

— Adapted from *Games Stages and Assessment,* Belka (2007), National Association for Sport and Physical Education.

Stage 3 of the games stages assessment examines competitive play in small-sided games, with a few targeted tactics. Assessments in Stage 3 should focus on the few targeted tactics and on how well the players assist each other, use their emotions in a positive manner and display appropriate sportsmanship. See Figure 4.4, which can help teachers analyze components of play on offense and defense.

Figure 4.4. Sample On- and Off-the-Ball Soccer Assessment

Player Observation Worksheet: Record the number of times each occurs.

Player/Team: _____ Observer: _____

Off-the-Ball Activity		On-the-Ball Activity	
Number of times that the player:		Number of times that the player:	
Is open in a good position to receive the ball	_____	Challenges the opponent's ball and interferes with timing, or more	_____
Calls in a good position to receive the ball	_____	Has a quality first touch to control the ball	_____
Calls in a weak position to receive the ball	_____	Makes a quality pass to a teammate	_____
Is in a good position to support the defense	_____	Dribbles the ball in control for two or more meters	_____
Is in a good position to support an offensive move	_____	Shoots on goal when open and has a good chance to score	_____
Total	_____	**Total**	_____

Mark a simple line for each occurrence and sum the totals for each item. Discuss this in relation to previous performance.

Identify Strengths:

Areas for Improvement Compared to Previous Play:

— Adapted from Huball & Robertson (April 2004), *Journal of Physical Education, Recreation and Dance*, American Alliance for Health, Physical Education, Recreation and Dance.

Stage 3 assessment lends itself to children with disabilities, because it progresses with extensions from 1 v 1 to 2 v 2 to 3 v. 3, etc. For example, teachers can assess children with autism on basketball offense and defense using a 1 v 1 situation, and can assess other students in the class using a 2 v 2 or a 3 v 3 scenario. As players are added, teachers have to determine what size playing area and what type of equipment to use, as well as any restrictions on players' movement within part or the entire playing space. For example, students who are distracted easily benefit from being assessed in a smaller playing area. Teachers can make those types of decisions as part of the general curriculum, with learners' attributes in mind (*Figure 4.5*).

Teachers can use the assessment in Figure 4.5 for many different sports and games. When children with disabilities are involved, the UDL approach can help ensure that the modifications that are necessary are documented as part of the assessment. The UDL approach accounts for skill abilities within the class, as well as the learners' attributes. With that in mind, teachers can modify the level of rules, types of equipment, class set-up (e.g., large groups, small groups, dyads) and level-of-play difficulty to meet children's needs within the class.

Using Figure 4.5, for example, a student with cerebral palsy might benefit from using a weighted or heavy ball, a student with low vision or ADD might benefit from using a bright ball, a student who has poor eye/hand coordination might benefit from using a slightly deflated ball and a student with autism might benefit from using a textured ball.

Teachers also can break the class into groups that lend themselves well to the games stage level being taught. Keep in mind that all children will be assessed with the same evaluation, but the assessments will document modifications to the game situation.

Figure 4.5. Sample Stage 3 for Volleyball (Stand-Up or Sit Volleyball)

5 = Nearly all the time.
4 = 70 percent to 80 percent of the time.
3 = 40 percent to 60 percent of the time.
2 = 20 percent to 30 percent of the time.
1 = Rarely, if ever; student might not even know.

Name	Bump	Set	Serve	Moves to space
Jeremy P.	4	5	4	3
Chloe A.	3	4	3	4
Miso J.	3	2	3	3
Ariel H.	4	5	5	5
Pierre D.	3	4	3	2
Justin H.	3	5	4	3
Mario Q.	3	5	5	4
Anrdea B.	4	5	5	4
Helen W.	2	3	2	2

Comments related to specific children:

Miso uses a beach ball and serves closer to the net.

Justin uses a trained peer tutor for every class.

In *Games Stages and Assessment,* Belka suggests using modified balls, goals, environment and rules, as well as simplifying games that are too complex. That's particularly important for children who have difficulty moving (e.g., those with cerebral palsy) and students who have difficulty remembering the sequence of actions and appropriate responses (e.g., those with cognitive delays). We've provided an example of a variety of possible game modifications for basketball in Figure 4.6 below.

Figure 4.6. Possible Game Modifications for Basketball

Equipment	Rules	Environment	Instruction
Basketball	Increase number of fouls allowed	Cones as boundaries	Verbal cues
Large ball	No three-second rule	Bright boundaries	Demonstration/Model
Small ball	No double-dribble rule	Ropes as boundaries	Physical assistance
Bright ball	Can walk with ball without dribbling	Beeper/Auditory boundaries	Peer tutor
Textured ball	Different points a warded for baskets	Visual shooting line	Paraeducator
Heavy ball	Extra step on lay-up	Smooth surface	Task cards (enlarged if needed)
Light ball	Undefended	Modify court size	Pictures
Foam ball (Easy to grip)	No defense for X number of seconds	Stations	Tactile modeling
Nerf® ball (Students will be less afraid of being hit)	Free shooting (no defense)	Number of players	Guided discovery
Beach ball	Everyone touches ball before a shot is attempted		Problem solving
Deflated ball (easier to grip and does not roll far)	Pass X number of times before a shot is attempted		Task analysis
Auditory ball (good for students who are visually impaired or have ADD/ADHD	Vary playing times		Proximity (instructor stands close to target student/students)
Buzzer basket	Limit boundaries		Interpreter
High basket	Small-sided games (i.e., 3 v 3)		Individualized instruction (1:1)
Low basket	Increase number of players		Sign language
Bright basket			Feedback
Wide basket			

— Adapted, with permission, from *Strategies for Inclusion: A Handbook for Physical Educators,* Lieberman & Houston-Wilson (2009), Human Kinetics.

The modifications offered in Figure 4.6 are only suggestions; teachers can try whatever might work and document on the assessment accommodations that benefit the child. For example, if a child is learning passing and catching skills, using a smaller ball, a bounce-pass and a peer tutor would be documented on the assessment and can be added to the child's IEP.

Referring to the UDL concept; the teacher would look at the class skills and attributes, the function of the child with the disability, and the objective of the sport and level of the sport being taught. Let's say the teacher is teaching basketball and the class is a 3rd-grade class. A child named Jose uses a walker and can dribble but has to stop to dribble. They are learning dribbling, passing and pivoting. The above modifications of equipment, space and rules would be considered. For this unit, Jose's skills could be assessed while playing small-sided games. The ball could be a regulation-size ball; he could play undefended; he could pivot by planting his walker, turning his feet, then moving his walker; he could use a peer tutor, if desired, to help him get the ball; and he would have an unlimited amount of time to pass the ball to his defended peers. This way, the class is still working on the objectives and Jose can be assessed on the same objectives within his abilities, with a peer to support him. Everyone can be assessed using Level 3 of this assessment.

Responsible personal and social behavior is another component of Stage 3 assessment. All children, regardless of disability, should be able to display responsible behavior, encouragement to others and sportsmanship. In some instances, they might need prompting, modeling and even scripts to help facilitate the behavior, but it's a required component of game assessments.

Similar to Stage 3, **Stage 4** consists of a more in-depth assessment with regard to game complexity and tactics; therefore, it falls outside the scope of this book. Although, typically, Stage 4 applies to students in middle or high school, teachers can use the ideas that follow with upper-elementary (4th & 5th) grades.

Disability Sport as Part of the Games Stages Assessment

Of course, one can use games stage concepts for disability sports: those that mirror able-bodied sports but are played by athletes with disabilities. Some examples: sit volleyball, wheelchair rugby, wheelchair basketball, wheelchair tennis, goal ball (for those with visual impairments), wheelchair soccer, wheelchair slalom racing and swimming without using the legs. Teachers can use the same assessment concepts for these sports, which can provide wonderful tools to aid in disability awareness.

Example: Lucas is a 6th-grader with a spinal cord injury. He uses a wheelchair, and his class is working on volleyball. As part of the unit, Lucas's teacher has the class watch the 2008 Paralympics sitting volleyball championship game on You Tube. The class then plays sitting volleyball on two courts for the next two weeks. Lucas is included completely as the class played sit volleyball, because he can participate fully. The teacher uses a games assessment modified for stand-up or sit volleyball, and all the children are challenged and have fun.

Summary

Games stages build on themselves, from simple to complex. A child must learn the skills in Stage 1 before he/she can implement them in Stages 2 & 3. The modifications used in the assessments in game Stage 1 can be used throughout a unit. Harold, for example, is a dwarf. He uses the modification of an underhand shot in basketball, because it's easier on his shoulders and he can throw it higher than an overhand shot. He uses this modification consistently for each game stage. As children move through their elementary years, the modifications become accepted practice, and peers grow accustomed to accommodating the unique needs of their classmates.

This chapter provided examples of each games stage, with sample modifications for a variety of children with different disabilities. It's up to the teacher, the paraeducators, peers and the child him/herself to ensure that each unit is assessed, and that all children continue to improve on all aspects of game play. With some creativity and patience, anything is possible.

CHAPTER 5

Establishing Criteria for Assessments

Lauren J. Lieberman, Ph.D.
The College at Brockport, State University of New York

Jacalyn Lea Lund, Ph.D.
Georgia State University

Why Set Criteria for Students?

One of the most important parts of an assessment is the criterion that the teacher uses for determining whether a student has achieved success. With written tests, a teacher might use a percentage of correct responses as the criterion for performance (e.g., 70 percent and above is passing/acceptable). A psychomotor-skill test criterion might require students to perform a skill three times consecutively while using correct form or to hold a balance for five seconds. Teachers also can communicate criteria through rubrics and scoring guides.

This chapter is written to complement the NASPE Assessment Series book *Creating Rubrics for Physical Education* (Lund, 2000), which explains the use of rubrics in the assessment process and the benefits of using them. The purpose of this chapter is to ensure that teachers understand how to create and use these scoring guides and rubrics with all children, including those with disabilities.

What Are Rubrics?

Put simply, rubrics articulate the criteria or standards that teachers use to evaluate student work. They help clarify what teachers consider important and tell students exactly how assignments/assessments will be evaluated and/or graded (Lund, 2000). By reading the rubrics, students know the "rules" regulating the assessment or assignment. A good rubric reveals to the teacher and the student the degree to which the student met the instruction objective(s).

Typically, rubrics are complex and require the scorer to make a judgment about the level of quality that the student has displayed regarding the performance or product. Analytic rubrics allow the scorer to rate the quality of the performance. Performance lists allow the assessor only to note whether the student demonstrated the skill or performance, or not. Analytic rubrics allow the assessor the opportunity to indicate the rudimentary presence of a trait or characteristic.

Some assessments need a less complex scoring guide than a rubric. Checklists and point-system scoring guides are performance lists that require users to decide whether a trait or characteristic is present or not. They consist of a list of descriptors that the scorer can mark to indicate the presence of the characteristic. Whereas all traits on a checklist have equal value, teachers can indicate that a trait is more important than another, or they can give it more weight by assigning a point value to the item.

Rubrics and performance lists can help improve learning for all students when they articulate the criteria used for the assessment clearly, and the criteria are observable and measurable. Because students know the criteria, they no longer need to depend on just the teacher for feedback. Students can learn to evaluate their peers' performance and achievement critically. Also, students can self-assess, note their current level of achievement and work to improve. This process proves to be quite motivational, because students know when they have achieved mastery or success. And using scoring guides in classes that include children with disabilities also yields many benefits, including the following:

1. Teachers can include a spectrum of skill-level expectations on the rubric so that they can evaluate each child using the rubrics or performance lists, and each child can feel that he/she is a part of the class.

2. Teachers can measure each child's objective continuously throughout the unit to guide future instruction.

3. All students can work individually, with partners or in a small group, so that teachers can record their progress during the class.

4. Students can take the scoring guide home and practice individual skills for homework.

5. The level of support or physical assistance that children with disabilities need can be indicated, thus providing documentation for use in future classes or for legal purposes.

6. Teachers can include rubrics or performance lists on students' IEPs to indicate achievement expectations.

Although creating separate rubrics for students with disabilities can prove time-consuming, in many cases, teachers can use the rubrics for several years, as students progress through the program. If the rubric notes the level of assistance or support that each child needs, it allows the teacher to demonstrate student learning that results from participating in a program. Also, when students see such evidence of their progress, it provides motivation and incentive to work hard.

Knowing Where to Set the Bar

Assessment's primary purpose should be to enhance student learning. When students are learning new skills, an assessment can determine whether the student has mastered each new skill or concept, or whether more practice or instruction is necessary. The criteria established for the assessment set the bar for achievement. One can approach setting the criteria in two ways.

First, if the goal is to have students reach a level of proficiency high enough to play the game at a recreational level (e.g., having fun with their friends), then set the criteria at a level that will allow them to eventually succeed (e.g., be able to play at that level).

The second approach might be necessary when working with students who have disabilities, as it sometimes is simply not realistic to expect a recreational level of competence given the time available or the child's abilities. But, with modifications, it's possible for them to enjoy success. The teacher must modify the criteria for the class using a level of achievement appropriate for each individual child. This approach ensures that all students can maximize their potential and become physically educated. But teachers must make the criteria modification as early as possible to comply with the UDL approach explained in Chapter 1.

When setting the bar for students with disabilities, the teacher must keep the needs of the individual student in the forefront. A scoring guide can cover a wide range of abilities and disabilities and can accommodate heterogeneous classes with relatively minor changes. If a student has asthma, for example, no accommodation is necessary for the cognitive or affective domain criteria, but accommodation probably is necessary for psychomotor skills that involve cardiorespiratory endurance. Similarly, children with emotional disabilities might not need accommodation for psychomotor skills, but they might need different criteria for the affective domain.

Rubrics and performance lists can be written for a variety of levels, and can describe quantitative or qualitative attributes or address process and product elements. Criteria for assessments typically are used to assess the *process* or quality of a movement skill (e.g., correct form, critical elements) or the *product* or quantity of a movement skill (e.g., how far, how fast, how many).

When writing criteria, teachers must remember that the *parameter* — or the conditions under which the movement skill was performed — is important and should be stated. When establishing criteria for children with disabilities, teachers must remember that parameter is often a significant modifier, because a variety of conditions can be used. Examples of parameters might include using physical assistance (e.g., walker for support, physical guidance), equipment modifications (e.g., beeper ball, balls that are slightly deflated, lowered nets, using a batting tee), or space modifications (larger or smaller, depending on the activity).

Developing Rubrics for Students With Disabilities

When children with disabilities are included in general physical education classes, teachers can take one of two approaches for developing rubrics. The first is to enhance an existing scoring guide or rubric to accommodate a wider variety of student skills. For example, teachers might need to modify rubrics developed for typically developing students to allow students with disabilities to be included in the assessment.

Example: A 3rd-grade curriculum included a jump-rope rubric that listed three levels: red, white and blue. For the red, or basic, level, students had to be able to jump rope at a proficient level to even qualify. So, teachers added green and yellow (school colors) levels to accommodate students who were emerging jumpers.

The second approach is to develop a new set of criteria for the assessment, written exclusively for students with disabilities.

Enhancing Existing Scoring Guides or Rubrics

Instead of developing an entirely new set of criteria, it might be possible to alter existing scoring guides to accommodate students with disabilities. Some suggestions for doing so follow. With all modifications, it's important that teachers leave space for comments to indicate which, if any, modifications were used for each child.

Extension enhancement. Sometimes, a rubric starts too high for a child with a disability or too low for a highly skilled student. The concept of rubric extensions allows for more levels of criteria within a given activity. For example, teachers made a dribbling rubric for a 7th-grade class as shown in Figure 5.0.

Figure 5.0. Example of Extending a Progressive Checklist With Dribbling for a Typically Developing Child

Dribbling Progressive Checklist

Level 1	Dribbles at waist level with fingertips, using right and left hands, 20 times each hand.
Level II	Dribbles at waist level with fingertips, using right and left hands, 30 times each hand.
Level III	Dribbles at waist level with fingertips, using right and left hands, 20 times each hand, while walking.
Level IV	Dribbles at waist level with fingertips, using right and left hands, 20 times each side of the body, while jogging around the gym.

Dribbling Checklist With Extensions

Level I	Dribbles with one hand 10 times while sitting on the ground.
Level II	Dribbles with two hands while sitting in a chair.
	Dribbles from right to left while sitting in a chair.
Level III	Dribbles at waist level, with right and left hands, 20 times each hand.
	Dribbles at waist level using fingertips, with right and left hands, 20 times each hand.
Level IV	Dribbles at waist level with fingertips, using right and left hands, 30 times each hand.
Level V	Dribbles at waist level with fingertips, using right and left hands, 20 times each hand, while walking.
Level VI	Dribbles at waist level with fingertips, using right and left hands, 20 times each hand, while jogging around the gym.

Analytic rubric. Figure 5.1 on the following page provides an example of a modification of a quantitative rubric. Note that it allows the scorer to indicate that the performer can demonstrate the skill some of the time, which is different from the single level of performance required for performance list scoring guides.

Inset within a rubric. Some students with disabilities will be able to master most of the criteria on a rubric developed for typical children, but teachers might need to add an inset *(Figure 5.2)* to satisfy a requirement on an IEP. In some cases, that might mean that a child with a disability will be working on a modification to one of the traits or characteristics on the class rubric while adhering to the criteria established for the class on the rest of the rubric. In other words, one rubric is in place for the entire class, and another rubric specific to the student's IEP goals is embedded within that rubric. This inset approach means that the student with a disability can be working on the overall class objective through the class rubric, as well as on his/her IEP goals through criteria that is unique for that child.

Example: Sam is a 7th-grader with Down syndrome who has low physical endurance. To enhance his endurance, the teacher created an inset rubric that leads him toward working on keeping his heart rate in the target zone for three sets of six minutes per class. By having the inset rubric incorporated into the existing class

(Continued on p. 47)

Figure 5.1. Sample Technique Assessment for Tennis Skills

Name: _____

Check to indicate which of the following critical elements are present.
I = Independently   **PPA** = Partial physical assistance   **TPA** = Total physical assistance

		Level of Assistance	Occasionally (Success 25% of the time)	Sometimes (Success 50% of the time)	Consistently (3 times in a row)
Forehand	Ready position				
	Moves to the ball				
	Shoulders turned and perpendicular				
	Early racquet preparation				
	Steps into the shot				
	Low-to-high stroking motion				
Backhand	Ready position				
	Moves to the ball				
	Shoulders turned and perpendicular				
	Early racquet preparation				
	Steps into the shot				
	Low-to-high stroking motion				
Serve	Readyposition				
	Toss				
	Little circle				
	Point of contact				
	Follow-through & finish				
Forehand volley	Ready position Racquet & shoulder turn				
	Steps toward ball				
	Forward motion of the racquet				
	Racquet hand above the wrist				
	Follow-through				

Figure 5.2. Sample Inset Rubric for Soccer Game Play

Name: _____ Date: _____

Classroom Teacher: _____ File Color: _____ No: ____

Skills	1	2	3	4
Player Position	Stands in one place; rarely moves to an open position or moves randomly on the field of play.	Moves to an area covered by opposing team.	Usually moves to be in open area; makes adjustments when he/she sees that the ball is coming.	Constantly moves to an open position; is always ready to receive a pass; moves to areas away from other teammates.
Ball/Puck Control	Loses the ball when dribbling.	Maintains control of the ball when moving slowly.	Maintains control of the ball when dribbling.	Always maintains control of the ball when dribbling; skills are automatic and effortless.
CV Fitness ** Sam's inset (*See next page*)	Must stop often to rest; is unable to move the length of the field.	Can stay even with play for about half the length of the field. Stops to rest are short and allow the player to get back into the action.	Is able to move continuously with the ball, regardless of the distance traveled. Can stay even with play during the duration of play.	Sprints to reach the ball; often is the first person to reach a ball. Is able to pace self so that he/she moves continuously. Appears to move tirelessly throughout the entire game, regardless of the amount of minutes played.
Rules	Violates rules and thinks that they were made for others.	Displays frequent lack of knowledge of rules.	Displays knowledge of most rules.	Always displays knowledge of rules.
Safety	Play is out of control and unsafe.	Play might endanger others' safety, but not done deliberately.	Plays safely with the exception of an occasional (one or two per game) infraction.	Plays safely; encourages safe behavior by others.
Etiquette	Impolite to classmates; makes rude comments and/or plays.	Might try to cheat; plays only to win.	Shows good sports etiquette; is considerate of others.	Compliments teammates and opponents on good plays.

Figure 5.2. *(Cont.)*

** Indicate the amount of time that Sam can move continuously during a game with spoken encouragement.

	1 minute	2 minutes	3 minutes	4 minutes	5 minutes	6 minutes
Set 1						
Set 2						
Set 3						

(Continued from p. 44)

rubric during a soccer unit, Sam can participate in a class game and will be encouraged to participate in play for intervals of six minutes. In that way, he meets his individual endurance goal while participating in the class unit.

An example of Sam's rubric can be a simple way to indicate the amount of time for each episode.

The teacher can fill out a rubric for Sam each class or each week.

Developing Independent Criteria for Assessments for Students With Disabilities

For some students with disabilities, the most prudent decision is to develop a scoring guide or rubric for the activity being taught. The Scooter Traveler rubric presented in Figure 5.3 on the following page provides an example of a progressive skill checklist. The checklist includes a progression of skills, and the teacher or students can indicate which skills the child has mastered. In addition, this rubric allows the instructor to indicate the levels of assistance that a student needs to attain each objective.

Task-analysis checklist. In some cases, children with disabilities might need a skill to be further task-analyzed for them to put all of its parts together (Block, Lieberman & Conner-Kuntz, 1998). With a task-analysis checklist, teachers can task-analyze the skills into very small parts to detect a child's progress and to teach the skill's component parts. Figure 5.4 provides an example of a rubric analysis.

Individual rubric. Children with special needs might require rubrics developed specifically for their individual needs. Although a child might be able to participate in a particular unit of instruction (e.g., dance), he/she might work specifically on balance while the rest of the class works on mastering a variety of dance steps. The child with limited balance who is engaged in a dance unit can work on toe-walking for distance, standing on one foot for a certain length of time and challenging equilibrium without losing balance. The child's individual rubric would reflect those skills and his/her ability to perform them. This individual rubric is entirely separate from the class rubric. The child would perform with his/her class, yet use different assessment criteria.

(Continued on p. 50)

Figure 5.3. Scooter Traveler

Instructions: Mark the appropriate box when the student performs the task at each level of assistance.

√ = No assistance needed   PA = Partial assistance needed   TA = Total assistance needed

Student Name: **Date Accomplished:**

Level	Description of Skill	Total Assistance	Partial Assistance	No Assistance
Slick Rider	Student lies on scooter while teacher, aide or peer pulls/pushes across gym, 1 time.			
Hammer Hold	Student sits or lies on scooter and holds a hula hoop or jump rope. Teacher, aide or peer grasps the other end of hoop or rope and pulls the student across the gym, 1 time.			
Speed-ster	Student sits on scooter and pushes self across gym with legs, demonstrating control, 1 time. Student lies on scooter and pulls self across gym with arms, demonstrating control, 1 time.			
Road-runner	Student sits on scooter and pushes self across gym 50 feet with the legs, demonstrating control, 2 times consecutively.			
	Student lies on scooter and pulls self 50 feet with arms, demonstrating control, 2 times consecutively. Student lies on scooter while teacher, aide or peer pulls the student 50 feet 2 times. Student sits or lies on scooter and holds a hula hoop or jump rope. Teacher, aide or peer grasps the other end of hoop or rope and pulls the student 50 feet, 2 times.			
Quick-silver	Student sits on scooter and pushes self across gym with the legs, demonstrating control, 5 times.			
	Student lies on scooter and pulls self across gym with arms, demonstrating control, 5 times.			
	Student lies on scooter while teacher, aide or peer pulls across the gym 5 times.			
	Student sits or lies on scooter and holds a hula hoop or jump rope. Teacher, aide or peer grasps the other end of hoop or rope and pulls the student across the gym 5 times.			
Blast-Off	Student sits on scooter and pushes self across gym with arms and legs, demonstrating control, 5 times.			

Sitting: _____   Standing: _____

Comments:

Note: Teacher must indicate whether the child is lying down or sitting. Also, the child can work on several different **levels** during one class or unit.

Figure 5.4. Skill Analysis Checklist for Foul-Shooting

I = Independent   PA = Partial assistance   TA = Total assistance   Demo = Demonstration

Student Name:

Level	Description of skill	I	PA	TA	Demo
Minnesota Lynx	• Knees bent				
Charlotte Sting	• Knees bent				
	• Eyes on basket				
Cleveland Rocker	• Knees bent				
	• Eyes on basket				
	• Body extends upward				
New York Liberty	• Knees bent				
	• Eyes on basket				
	• Body extends upward				
	• Correct hand position on ball a. Non-shooting hand supports ball held in shooting hand b. Shooting hand is palm-up, fingers facing shooter c. Wrist flexed forward				
Houston Comet	• Knees bent				
	• Eyes on basket				
	• Body extends upward				
	• Correct hand position on ball a. Non-shooting hand supports ball held in shooting hand b. Shooting hand is palm-up, fingers facing shooter c. Wrist flexed forward				
	• Shooting arm extends up & forward				
	• Follow through by extending arm fully toward basket & reaching with shooting hand				

Picture rubric. Teachers can develop a picture calendar rubric using the Boardmaker® programs and follow the criteria that students are working on. The teacher can work with the special education teacher, speech therapist or paraeducator to ensure that it's clear to the student.

Using the batting example from the symbols pictured at right, the teacher could show the picture of batting, demonstrate batting and say "Your turn" to the child. If the student needs to try it five times, the teacher can show the number "5" and then show how many at-bats the child has remaining.

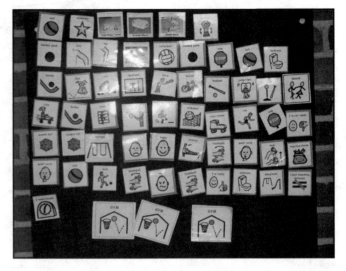

Specific Adaptations to Individual Rubrics

In addition to those general adaptations to rubrics, teachers must address some adaptations related to specific disabilities when developing individual rubrics. This section will provide a brief overview of some ideas to accommodate those disabilities.

Physical disabilities. Children with physical disabilities can benefit from performing the rubric level from a wheelchair, using a walker or with their orthotics. Teachers should emphasize the elements of the rubric that the child can perform. If needed, the teacher can add further description to the rubric levels — within each level or at the end of the rubric — to accommodate a child in a wheelchair.

Cognitive/learning disabilities. Children with cognitive or learning disabilities will benefit from pictures and demonstrations of the different rubric levels. Most helpful: highlighting numbers or levels. Teacher should provide a clear review and feedback on where the child is on the rubric and what he/she has to do to reach the next level.

Emotional disorders. Rubrics are especially good for children with emotional disorders, because expectations for the child are stated ahead of time. In addition, the students can rewrite the rubric in their own words (*see No. 8 on p. 53*). The skills will be at their level, and they can challenge themselves further. To minimize any frustration or issues with performance, teachers should ensure that the rubrics are specific to each child's ability. And teachers should discuss expectations and set goals with each student who writes his/her own rubric.

Pervasive developmental disorders. Children with pervasive developmental disorders will benefit from picture symbols or object symbols for each level with numbers. Teachers often can embed the symbols into students' picture calendars.

Creating Rubrics to Include Everyone

Retrofitting an existing rubric or performance list to fit a class with children with disabilities can be time-consuming but rewarding. And creating scoring guides that include everyone is the key to using a UDL approach. We offer the following suggestions so that teachers can use appropriate criteria to help all children learn.

1. Develop a rubric for the class.

A good scoring guide should help all students become more skillful, more knowledgeable or to behave in an acceptable manner. It should be challenging to each member of the class, including those at the highest and lowest levels of performance. Including a level to accommodate even the most novice performers will help them determine where they are with their skills and what they must do to move to the next level.

It's important to start with simple skills and use easy-to-understand terms with observable and measurable descriptors. If the rubric is written correctly, the highest performers will continue to be challenged, even in a heterogeneous class. Regarding psychomotor skills, some students who have not been diagnosed with special-needs delayed motor skills also can benefit from an expanded rubric with a simpler entry point. In the rubric seen in Figure 5.5, several students had to start at the Gymnast level but could move up the rubric with some practice and support.

2. Align criteria to the class objective.

Skill descriptors should focus on class objectives. *Example:* You're creating a rubric for the balance beam and you must ensure that every child in your 4th-grade class is challenged and can focus on improving his/her skills on this part of your gymnastics unit. Your objective is balance, motor skill development and changing levels. Two students in your class are overweight and have difficulty with balance. One student has Down syndrome and has a wide base stance and difficulty with balance. For this class, the lowest level of performance requires students to walk a one-foot-wide line on the floor the equivalent to the length of a balance beam. At this level, students can succeed and can practice the skills related to the objective for the class without fear. See Figure 5.5 for an example.

3. Place small increments between levels.

The increments of difficulty between skills should be small enough that most students would be able to move up at least one level to another within the unit's timeframe. When working with a diverse class, the rubric used as a formative assessment should have small increments between levels so that students — with practice and study — will be able to progress to the next level. Teachers must be careful, though, when writing these levels to ensure that the difference between levels is identifiable. Figure 5.5 provides an example of a progressive rubric, in which students can see clearly what they must do to progress to the next level of difficulty.

4. Use clear descriptions in the rubric so that it's clear when a child meets that level.

The quality of how well each child performs the skill, how many times and what level of support should be clear within the criteria. Figure 5.5 specifies the direction of travel, the number of repetitions and the level of support. If the information is specific enough, each child's current level of performance can be taken right from the rubric and placed into his/her IEP.

5. Leave room for comments.

When developing criteria for assessing all students, it's a good idea to leave room for comments. When assessing students with disabilities, it's essential. Comments can give parents, administrators, paraeducators and future teachers valuable information about how students performed on class assessments.

Figure 5.5. Balance Beam Gymnastics Rubric

Instructions: Mark the appropriate box when the student performs the task at each level of assistance.

√ = No assistance needed   PA = Partial assistance needed   TA = Total assistance needed

Level	Element	Level of Support		Comments
Gymnast	Walk forward across the line 1 – 3 times.	With Assistance	Without Support	
	Floor / Low beam / High beam			
Honorable Mention	Walk forward or sideways across the line 3 times.			
	Floor / Low beam / High beam			
Bronze Medalist	Walk backward across the line 1 – 3 times.			
	Floor / Low beam / High beam			
Silver Medalist	Walk forward or backward across the line 1 – 3 times while changing levels 3 times.			
	Floor / Low beam / High beam			
Gold Medalist	Leap forward across the line 1 – 3.			
	Floor / Low beam / High beam			
Championship Gymnast	Complete a forward roll across the line 2 times consecutively without falling.			
	Floor / Low beam / High beam			
Olympian Gymnast	Complete a cartwheel across the line 2 times consecutively without falling.	Low beam	High beam	
	Floor / Low beam / High beam			
Gymnastics Instructor	Teach 1-3 students how to perform any of the above skills on the beam.			

Example: Aiden has autism and performs much better when music is playing during class because he is more focused and happier. Putting that information in the comments section makes Aiden's teacher next year aware of the accommodation.

Example: Josie uses a wheelchair, but can walk with her walker. She performed at the Championship level with her walker and a peer tutor to help her. Putting that information in the comments section made it clear how Josie succeeded.

6. Incorporate a level to recognize peer support.

It's a good idea to allow a rubric level at the top so that higher-skilled students can get credit for supporting or helping students who are still learning. Once a student has reached the Olympian Gymnast level *(Figure 5.5)*, he/she can turn to others, help them improve and earn credit for that.

7. Include pictures and/or videos as exemplars.

Students with and without disabilities will benefit from photos and videos of certain skills. Seeing what students have done in the past is an excellent way to facilitate learning. Students will see a visual interpretation of the criteria and have a clearer idea of what's expected of them.

8. Allow students the opportunity to rewrite rubrics into their own words.

The first part of this chapter stated that the first purpose of assessment should be to enhance student learning. Allowing students to rewrite a rubric using their own words is an excellent way to help them understand expectations for learning. We're not suggesting that teachers should allow students to create their own rubrics; setting the criteria for performance and determining expectations for learning is the teacher's responsibility. But allowing students to rewrite established criteria often leads to questions, helps them clarify what certain words mean and provides a way to increase their comprehension of those expectations.

Summary

Establishing the criteria for achievement is important when assessing all children. Criteria are conveyed to students easily using scoring guides that are thorough and comprehensive. The primary purpose of assessment is to enhance learning. Using high-quality rubrics and performance lists are natural ways for teachers to assess each child's ability. Through some creativity, teamwork and planning, all children can be challenged, can improve their performance and can reach their potential.

CHAPTER 6

Assessing & Improving Fitness in Elementary Physical Education

Danielle Blanchard
Guilderland Central School District

John Foley, Ph.D.
State University of New York — Cortland

An increasing body of literature supports the importance of health-related fitness in reducing health disparities between children with and without disabilities. As such, it's vital that teachers assess components of students' health–related fitness, not only to set education goals and objectives but also to ensure that students are making progress toward those goals and objectives.

This chapter is intended to help readers assess the health-related fitness of all children in the elementary school setting and to complement ideas presented in the NASPE Assessment Series book *Assessing & Improving Fitness in Elementary Physical Education,* 2nd Edition (Strand & Mauch, 2008). The chapter will describe a variety of ideas to help teachers modify health-related assessments in assessing and improving fitness by using the UDL approach.

This chapter:

- Reviews aspects of health-related fitness assessment.

- Shares ways to infuse UDL into health-related fitness assessment.

- Provides examples of modifications for health-related fitness assessment and heart health activities.

Recent trends indicate that, during the elementary school years, it's more important to expose children to concepts of health-related fitness and less important to use that information for comparison and grading. That is seen in *The Brockport Fitness Test Manual* (Winnick & Short, 1999), which does not offer age-based criteria until age 10, and also in *Fitnessgram®/Activitygram® Reference Guide* (Meredith & Welk, 1999), where lap and time standards are not recommended in the aerobic capacity testing until age 10. Further, in some of the other components of *Fitnessgram,* such as the trunk lift and pull-up, the healthy zone criteria do not change from age 5 until after age 10.

That's not to suggest that elementary school teachers should not assess health-related fitness, only that they shouldn't rely too heavily on children's scores for evaluation. Elementary school is the ideal level at which to start weaving health-related fitness assessment into teaching. For physical educators, it's important to have a measure by which to gauge both the learning and performance of all students so that, as the children age, they will understand all aspects of assessing and maintaining their own fitness. Strand and Mauch (2008) stress that concept, while recommending that teachers focus fitness assessment on participation until children reach age 9.

Regardless of whether teachers select *Fitnessgram®*, the President's Challenge or another physical fitness battery, it's important that they understand that particular disabilities can affect movement modes, movement abilities and health-related physical fitness potential. For that reason, we recommend the *Brockport* test manual for helping to develop assessment protocol for assessing fitness in children with disabilities.

Many of the *Brockport Fitness* test's components parallel items found in *Fitnessgram®* and the President's Challenge, making the transition from one test to another almost seamless.

Health-related fitness is very important for children with disabilities. As America struggles with a childhood obesity crisis, little attention has been given to children with disabilities who have increased rates of obesity and lower physical activity levels than their peers without disabilities. Because of this health disparity between children with disabilities and their peers without disabilities, it's imperative that physical educators work toward improving health-related fitness for all children.

Using Paraeducators and Peer Tutors

In the general or inclusive physical education setting, paraeducators and peer tutors can play an important role in helping physical educators with all aspects of developing students' personal fitness profiles. It's imperative, though, that paraeducators and peer tutors are trained, with clear expectations for what they are supposed to do. Paraeducators or peer tutors can help with various aspects of the fitness assessment, as well as in setting goals and improvement strategies (Lieberman & Houston-Wilson, 2009). For example, they can help:

• Demonstrate necessary movements during fitness testing.

• Encourage and motivate students to complete an assessment.

• Serve as a "running buddy" alongside the student.

• Assist students with recording their own fitness scores.

Teachers who infuse the use of peer tutors into their classes are at an advantage because, with peer tutors comes the opportunity to provide students with multiple means of engagement. And a technique as simple as using a peer tutor to assist a student and provide greater detail of health-related fitness than what the teacher alone might otherwise be able to cover provides a great way to infuse the UDL approach into the physical education class.

Assessing Strength in Students With Physical Disabilities

This section reviews various ways to assess students with physical disabilities. These students might have cerebral palsy, paraplegia, quadriplegia, spina bifida or any other disability that impedes the use of their legs or arms or their motor function. They might move with a walker, crutches, a wheelchair or orthotic devices. When it comes to assessing strength, students with physical disabilities can participate in the same assessments as their peers, under the following modifications:

• Seated push-up from the wheelchair. The student places his/her hands on the armrest of the wheelchair and lifts the body until the arms are extended fully. Student repeats this as many times as possible.

- Isometric push-up. The student pushes up in the chair and holds the up position for as long as possible.

- Arm strength. Tie a Thera-Band® to a chair, wheelchair or permanent structure to assess the student's arm strength. The student then performs biceps curls, straight-arm lifts or triceps pulls. Use color of Thera-Band® and number of repetitions for assessment.

- Modified pull-up. Have the student lie on his/her back, with a bar set one to two inches above outstretched arms, with an elastic string stretched across seven to eight inches below bar to mark where the student is to pull up his/her chin. The student's feet can be on the ground or lifted up in the air with knees bent.

- Flexed-arm hang. From the pull-up position, chin above the bar, the student performs a flexed-arm hang for time. The time stops when the chin drops below the bar.

- Abdominal strength. The student completes a reverse curl — for which he/she pulls up the legs, instead of the upper torso, to contract the abdominals — while seated in his/her wheelchair.

Other *Brockport Physical Fitness Test Manual* (Winnick & Short, 1999) assessments for strength include those for an extended-arm hang, a dumbbell press, a wheelchair ramp test, a 40-meter push/walk and grip strength using a dynamometer.

Assessing Flexibility in Students With Physical Disabilities

Flexibility might be one of the most important components of fitness for students with cerebral palsy and spinal cord injuries. Students with cerebral palsy encounter restrictions in flexibility, especially when spasticity is prevalent. Also, hypertonicity of the muscles restricts range of motion in the joints.

Students with spinal cord injuries are susceptible to muscle imbalance resulting from their heavy reliance on the muscle groups that are working or innervated. Muscle imbalances around a joint will limit the range of motion of certain joint actions and reduce mobility. Many other disabilities create challenges for students to complete flexibility tests, as well. For students with limited range of motion and mobility, use comparable items from *The Brockport Physical Fitness Test Manual* (Winnick & Short, 1999), including the back-saver sit & reach, trunk lift, shoulder stretch, Modified Apley Test, Modified Thomas Test or Target Stretch Test. For complete scoring and additional assessments, see *The Brockport Physical Fitness Test Manual.*

Modified Apley Test. This test assesses mobility of the shoulder joint. Points are assigned for being able to touch the scapula, the top of the head and the mouth.

Modified Thomas Test. This test assesses the hip flexor. Lying supine on table, lift the left knee and pull it toward the chest with both hands. Measure how high the right leg lifts from the table surface. Repeat with the other leg.

Target Stretch Test. This test measures a student's maximum range of motion for a variety of joints, including the knee, wrist and elbow, as well as shoulder extension, shoulder abduction and external rotation, and forearm supination and pronation.

Assessing Cardiovascular Fitness in Students With Physical Disabilities

This section reviews the health-related fitness component of cardiovascular endurance for children with physical disabilities. One common measurement of cardiovascular fitness in adults is the heart rate. That makes it important for all children to learn how the heart rate is related to cardiovascular fitness. That said, because of the variability associated with growth during childhood, target heart rate based on adult equations are not recommended for children (Rowland, 2005). Further, children with spinal cord injuries might not be able to achieve certain heart rate intensities before fatiguing (Lockette & Keyes, 1994).

The Target Aerobic Movement Test (TAMT) is an assessment of aerobic functioning that allows flexibility in the activity chosen for the assessment (Winnick, 2005). TAMT is a good alternative when the mile run or the PACER (Progressive Aerobic Cardiovascular Endurance Run) tests are not an option.

Use a heart rate monitor during aerobic activity with the watch set so that it beeps only when the heart rate is above or below the set target zone. The target zone is set as about 70 percent to 85 percent of the working heart rate. The child then has to move enough to keep the heart rate between the parameters. TAMT measures the ability to exercise at or above a recommended target heart rate for 15 minutes (Winnick & Short, 2005).

Cognitive & Learning Disabilities

This section explores modifications that teachers can make to fitness items for children with cognitive or learning disabilities. Please note that teachers can use these modifications in addition to others recommended elsewhere in this chapter.

Suggested Modifications

- Use pictures in addition to spoken instructions for students with auditory processing deficits. The photos can be pictures of the child performing the activity or skill.

- Color-code and match fitness items set up in the gymnasium and on the child's personal fitness profile forms to assist processing and memory.

- Allow more time for a student with ADD or attention deficit hyperactivity disorder (ADHD) when giving directions. These students might need more time to process the information, and waiting a few minutes after instruction will allow them that time.

- Use a modified Borg Rate of Perceived Exertion Scale, which evaluates a student's perceived rate of exertion *(Figure 6.0)*. Using the Borg Scale, in combination with assessments of cardiovascular fitness, can help students with cognitive disabilities understand and assess their own fitness levels more accurately. Following the fitness assessment, students are asked to point to or express verbally the number (from one through 10) that best describes their level of exertion. By paring the fitness score with the perceived exertion, teachers can provide students with a concrete picture of how hard they are working.

- Use a paraeducator or peer tutor to run with students with disabilities or to help motivate them during assessment. *Example:* The peer can give the student a popsicle stick for each lap completed without stopping.

- Place a toy or picture in front of students who have problems pushing themselves to motivate them during the sit-and-reach test.

- Create portable picture strips that students can attach to a belt or pants leg and use as a guide to follow during an assessment. They can be single picture symbols or a stack of four or five skills strung together on a ring or carabiner.

- Use TAMT with students who are unable to monitor their own heart rates. Using a heart rate monitor during aerobic activity, the watch beeps only when the heart rate is above or below the set target zone. TAMT measures the ability to exercise at or above a recommended target heart rate for 15 minutes.

Figure 6.0. Modified Borg Rate of Perceived Exertion Scale

Rate of Perceived Exertion

🙂	1 2 3	Easy	
😐	4 5 6 7	Somewhat Hard	
😫	8 9 10	Hard	

Autism Spectrum Disorders

Because of the difficulty in communicating with children with autism, many of the ideas for assessing students with cognitive disabilities items can be very useful.

Suggested Modifications

- Color-code and match fitness items set up in the gymnasium and on the personal fitness profile forms.

- Use poly spots at each station to designate where the child is to stand or begin.

- Use the Borg Scale in combination with various fitness test items.

- Use communication picture boards, including these idea:

  - Use Velcro® flip books that children can use in the same way they use personal fitness booklets. Students can create picture strips that indicate what activity or component for which they plan to do the most work.

  - Create portable picture strips that students can attach to a belt or pants leg and use as a guide to follow during an assessment.

Sensory Impairments

This section reviews strategies to use for students who are visually impaired, blind, deaf or deaf/blind. The goal for each of these modifications is to assist impaired students' access to fitness testing with their peers.

Suggested Modifications

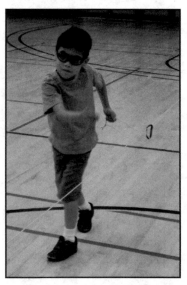

- Have a student with a visual impairment connected to a peer tutor with a short rope/tether during an assessment that involves running.

- Use a guide wire during assessments that involve running. A guide wire is a tight rope tied from one point to another about 100 to 300 feet apart. Use a carabiner with a short rope that slides across the long rope for the child to hold. Make sure that you have a different texture and a knot on the rope to warn the child when he/she is coming to the end (Lieberman, 2011).

- Allow the student — with assistance from a paraeducator or peer tutor — to create a personal fitness profile made of Velcro® strips.

- Use stationary exercises (e.g., rope jumping, stair climbing) to minimize having to maneuver through a space.

- Use a flashing light or arm motion for students who are hearing-impaired to indicate the "beep" during the PACER test.

Student using a guidewire to run a race.

Incorporating Health-Related Fitness Into Physical Education

Given the importance of health-related fitness, and the emerging evidence that moderate to vigorous physical activity plays a vital role in the health of students, it's essential that teachers introduce the fundamentals of cardiovascular fitness into physical education at an early age. The following provides ideas for using visual aids with circuit training, heart rate and grading by following the UDL approach to include students with disabilities.

One way to help children record their physical activity, for example, is by using the 60-minute-clock-based approach from the Strand & Mauch book *(Figure 6.1)*. Using visual aids, as this approach does, is particularly helpful for students with processing difficulties and with autism, because it provides a concrete reference.

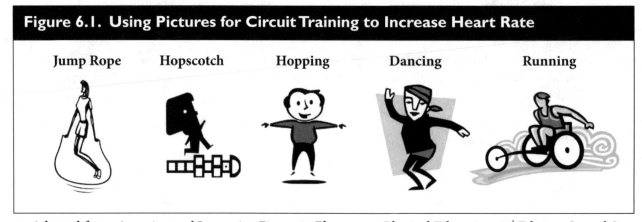

Figure 6.1. Using Pictures for Circuit Training to Increase Heart Rate

| Jump Rope | Hopscotch | Hopping | Dancing | Running |

— Adapted from *Assessing and Improving Fitness in Elementary Physical Education,* 2nd Edition, Strand & Mauch (2008), National Association for Sport and Physical Education.

Circuit Training

Circuit-training activities are excellent for students in the elementary grades and work on all body parts. With a few considerations using the UDL approach (*Figure 6.2*), all students can challenge themselves physically in the circuit. Figure 6.1, for example, demonstrates UDL by using pictures to give students ideas for circuit-training activities. In groups of four to six, students perform three to five minutes of the activity pictured at each station and then rotate to the next station in the circuit. Students record their heart rates or use the perceived exertion chart between each station.

Figure 6.2. The UDL Approach to Including All Children in Circuit Training	
Activity	**Variations**
Jumping rope	• Crawl, step or roll over a rope laid on the floor. • Jump side to side or forward and back over a rope tied to volleyball standards six inches above the floor. • Jump rope with no rope, just handles. • Bring the rope over the head and step over the rope.
Side-to-side jumping	• Jump over a line. • Step side to side. • Use the arms to raise the heart rate. • Push wheelchair forward and back.
Low rope/stationary jumps/vertical jumps	• Jump on mini-trampoline. • Jump on a mat. • Jump to a mark on a wall or hanging object. • Go up and down a ramp in a wheelchair or push forward and back on a mat.
Running in place	• Walk in place. • Wheel forward and back up a ramp or on a mat.
Hop on each foot	• Hop on each foot 3 times. • Hop from one poly spot to another. • Step side to side. • Push the wheelchair from one spot to another placed 3 feet apart.
Mutant hopscotch	• Step from one place to another. • Use visuals (e.g., poly spots, gym floor tape or signs taped to floor) for places to jump. • Push from one spot to another in your wheelchair.
Push-up variations	• Push-ups against a wall. • Kneeling push-ups. • Hold a push-up position and play games with balls, ropes dice, etc., in that position. • Wheelchair push-ups. • Wheelchair straight-arm hold for time.
Dance variations	• Use a streamer to emphasize motions, whether in a chair or not. • Dance using a hula hoop and move with different parts of the body. • Move at different levels. • Move with a partner. • Move within a certain space or within hula hoops. • Lie on a mat and move to music. • Sit or lie on a scooter board and move to the music.

Heart Rate

Students with disabilities can learn how to monitor their heart rates with their peers and record their heart rates on the pulse card *(Figure 6.3)*.

Figure 6.3. Pulse Card for Circuit Training

Name: _____ Homeroom: _____ My resting heart rate is: _____

Pulse Master (3 points)	Pulse Pro (2 points)	Pulse Pro (2 points)	Pulse Apprentice (1 point)
Finds pulse every time & records it on card.	Finds pulse & records it some of the time.	Finds pulse sometimes & records it.	Still trying to find the pulse.

Date	Pulse #1	Pulse #2	Pulse #3	Pulse #4		Rubric Score

— Reprinted from *Elementary Heart Health: Lessons & Assessments* (2001), Donna Baker, National Association for Sport and Physical Education.

Using the UDL approach will help students learn about and assess their heart rates. Here are a few suggestions:

- Have a trained peer tutor demonstrate and help the child find the pulse. The peer tutor can show the child how to take a pulse and walk him/her through the process. In this case, the peer tutor will also learn the skill better.

- Have a trained paraeducator demonstrate and help the child find the pulse. The paraeducator can show the child how to take the pulse and walk him/her through the process. The paraeducator also can lend support for the activities that the child undertakes to raise his/her heart rate.

- Task-analyze the skill of taking the pulse. Students can perform one or all of these steps, trying each time to improve their skills with determining the heart rate:

  o Find the pulse on the wrist or carotid artery.

  o Try to keep count for six seconds.

  o Practice recording the heart rate.

- If students are unable to take their own pulse rates, they could use a heart rate monitor worn on the chest, or use the less invasive electronic pulse device (i.e., Biosig Instruments' InstaPulse 201 wall-mount heart rate monitor). Rather than putting on a heart rate monitor, students simply go up to the unit mounted on the wall and grab the handle.

Summary

Health-related fitness is important for everyone. Students with disabilities might need variations in fitness circuits and assessments, but, with some careful planning, creativity and additional equipment, teachers can help every child improve his/her health-related fitness. This is the basis of UDL approach, which ensures all children the opportunity to benefit at the highest level from physical education class.

CHAPTER 7

Assessing Aquatics

Luis Columna, Ph.D.
Syracuse University

This chapter is intended to complement the NASPE Assessment Series book *Assessment of Swimming in Physical Education,* by Susan J. Grosse (2005), and presents ways to assess swimming ability in elementary physical education students with disabilities. The chapter covers the benefits and uses of assessment tools for swimming activities, as well as ways to develop and modify them.

Participating in a carefully designed aquatic intervention program, including pre-assessment, ongoing review of instruction and post-assessment, can yield remarkable improvement in the swimming skills of children with disabilities (Huettig & Darden-Melton, 2004). Aquatic experiences give children with disabilities a variety of opportunities that help them improve their well-being throughout life. Some of those improvements are related to aerobic capacity, strength and other functional skills that teachers can address through adapted aquatics.

"Adapted aquatics" refers to the adaptations to: instruction, equipment, strategies, strokes, swim skills, games, recreation skills, water-safety skills, and access to swimming instruction and recreation (Lepore, Gayle & Stevens, 2007). If teachers are to modify those areas, they need to identify tools for assessing students' performance. Teachers can use assessment results for many purposes, including to determine performance level and placement, and to assign grades, among others. Some of the goals are to collect as much information as possible for a child, so learning can be documented.

Preparing for Aquatic Assessment

Before identifying the performance level of a child with a disability in an aquatic environment, teachers should decide whether to use a formal assessment or to develop their own assessment based on the program/class's goals and objectives. The following section provides teachers with information on how to:

- Obtain information from parents/guardians and from the student with a disability.

- Select and modify existing assessment instruments.

- Conduct the assessment.

Obtaining the Child's Information

It's important for teachers to collect as much information as possible from the child's parents or guardians, either by interview (e.g., phone or in person) or by sending a survey/questionnaire home. Some of the information to gather: the child's disability, his/her preferred activities, family composition, communication preferences, etc. For example, understanding the child's behavior tendencies and/or how the child best communicates is valuable information to obtain from the parents and can save time during assessment and during instruction.

Teachers also can obtain information from the child him/herself or from other teachers. That might not be possible with all participants; but, when possible, it's a great way to gain understanding of a child's likes and dislikes. That way, the teacher will know the child's attributes. And knowing that will help the teacher apply the UDL approach as described in Chapter 1 for teaching and assessment purposes.

Figure 7.0. Example of Parent Questionnaire

Aquatics Parent Questionnaire

General Information • Y = Yes   N = No   NS = Not sure
(To help your child feel at ease)

_____ My child is comfortable in/loves the water.

_____ My child is afraid of the water.

_____ My child does not know how to swim and does not display a respectful understanding of the water.

_____ My child is able to put his/her face in the water.

_____ My child is **not** able to put his/her face in the water.

_____ My child is able to enter the water independently.

_____ My child is able to swim in shallow water.

_____ My child is able to swim in deep water.

Expressive Communication • Y = Yes   N = No   NS = Not sure

Primary Language: _____ English   _____ Spanish   _____Other: _____

_____ My child uses clear and understandable speech.

_____ My child talks in short sentences.

_____ My child talks in short phrases or uses single words.

_____ My child uses little spoken speech but uses gestures effectively.

_____ My child uses little or no functional speech.

_____ My child uses a communication board of communication cards/pictures.

_____ My child uses sign language. (If so, what signs does your child use?)

Figure 7.0. Example of Parent Questionnaire (Cont.)

Aquatics Parent Questionnaire

Receptive Communication • Y = Yes   N = No   NS = Not sure

_____ My child is able to follow complex (3-4 steps) directions.

_____ My child is able to follow simple verbal directions.

_____ My child talks in short phrases or uses single words.

_____ My child has little verbal speech but uses effective gestures.

_____ My child has little or no functional speech.

_____ My child uses a communication board of communication cards/pictures.

_____ My child uses sign language. If so, what signs does your child know and/or use?

Behavior • Y = Yes   N = No   NS = Not sure

_____ My child, generally, is cooperative and follows adult directions.

_____ My child requires minimal supervision to remain on task.

_____ My child needs constant supervision to stay on task.

_____ My child is distracted easily and has difficulty staying on task.

_____ My child might refuse to follow directions.

_____ My child might have a temper tantrum.

_____ **My child might become verbally and/or physically aggressive.**

** What type of incident(s) typically triggers the behavior?

Special Equipment • My child uses the following: (Please check all that apply.)

_____ Motorized or manual wheelchair

_____ Walker or crutches   * *Please note type:*

_____ Prosthesis   * *Please note location:*

_____ Braces   * *Please note location:*

_____ Hearing aid   * *Please circle type*:   <u>Ear</u>   <u>Body Pack</u>

_____ Ear plugs

_____ Protective helmet

_____ Corrective eyewear/glasses

Please share anything else you would like us to know about your child to help us provide the best possible experience.

When meeting with the student (or his/her parents), it's important to recognize individual differences, especially in terms of disabilities. That will help the teacher determine what modifications he/she needs to implement before assessing the child. As mentioned previously, one of the main reasons to assess students with disabilities is to determine their current levels of performance on different skills. No matter which assessment you use, it's important to include all children in the assessment.

After obtaining an overview of the child, the next steps are to determine what assessment tool to use and to conduct the assessment. Several factors will help with this task.

Because partnering with the parents is so valuable, the teacher needs to honor their expertise and desires. One parent might want his child to learn to swim because of safety concerns, while another parent might want her child to be involved in an aquatics program for the benefits of socializing with others.

The teacher's expertise is important, as well. Teachers need to be aware of the multiple benefits that a child with a disability can reap from being involved in an aquatics program. For that reason, it's important for teachers to share with parents/guardians what they believe to be the priorities for the child. Recommendations to parents might be to teach the child aquatics activities that the child can practice as a lifetime activity or to improve the child's overall health. Acknowledging parents' needs is vital to the assessment process because it can allow teachers to select the best assessment according to the child's ability and interests.

Selecting Assessments & Modifying Existing Instruments

This section presents examples of assessment tools that target the different learning domains: psychomotor, cognitive and affective. It also provides references to proven assessment tools. The ultimate intention here is to provide teachers with general ideas of how they can modify different existing assessment instruments to suit their programs' needs and help develop the child's IEP at the same time.

Assessment Instruments for Adapted Aquatics

Teachers can use a variety of assessment instruments to assess children with disabilities in aquatic environments (Bowerman, 2007; Humphries, 2008). Here are some tools for assessing the swimming abilities of children with disabilities:

1. **The Lone Star Adapted Aquatics Assessment Inventory and Curriculum** (LSAA) (Apache, Hisey & Blanchard, 2005). This is a checklist/basic rating scale that also provides instruction ideas and activities for each category. LSAA contains not only a curriculum, but an assessment inventory. The purpose of the assessment component is to assist instructors in determining and developing appropriate goals and objectives for each student (Lepore, Gayle & Stevens, 2007). It contains seven assessment levels, plus an initial assessment for placement and a safety assessment.

2. **Aquatic Readiness Assessment** (ARA) (Langendorfer & Bruya, 1995). This assessment instrument allows teachers to assess fundamental aquatic readiness skills that provide the foundation for all advanced aquatics skills, such as swimming strokes and diving.

3. **Developmental Aquatics Assessment** (Doremus, 1992). This instrument also allows teachers to assess fundamental readiness skills for very young children and those children with low cognitive functioning.

4. **Conatser Adapted Aquatics Screening Test.** This assessment tool provides normative data on the swimming abilities of children with different disabilities.

5. **Texas Woman's University Project Inspire Aquatic Assessment.** This curriculum-based assessment instrument addresses water-adjustment skills, flotation skills, basic propulsion and breathing, swimming stroke skills and entry and exit skills.

6. **Humphries Assessment of Aquatic Readiness (HAAR).** This assessment tool measures five phases in aquatics environments to assess children's swimming abilities: 1) mental adjustment; 2) introduction to water environment; 3) rotations; 4) balance and controlled movement; and 5) independent movement in the water.

Figure 7.1 provides a brief description of the components of each assessment instrument.

Figure 7.1. Components of Aquatic Assessments

	Water Orientation/ Adjustment	Water Entry/Exit	Breath Control	Buoyancy/ Floatation	Body Positioning	Arm Action	Leg Action	Combined Movement
LSAA	x	x	x	x	x	x	x	x
ARA	x	x	x	x	x	x	x	x
Project Inspire	x	x	x	x		x	x	x
Conatser	x	x	x	x		x	x	
Developmental Aquatics Assessment	x	x	x	x		x	x	
HAAR	x	x		x		x	x	x
	Different Levels (Beginning to Advanced)	Aligned Curriculum/ Activities	Initial Screen Test	Validity	Reliability	Safety		
LSAA	x	x	x	x	x	x		
ARA	x	x		x				
Project Inspire	x							
Conatser								
Developmental Aquatics Assessment								
HAAR		x		x	x	x		

— Adapted from "Assessment in Adapted Aquatics" (2007), Stephanie Bowerman, Texas Woman's University. Used with permission.

Conducting the Assessment

Once the teacher is familiar with the assessment tools he/she wants to use, the next step is to identify the learning domain to assess. A quality adapted aquatic program should provide activities that stimulate all learning domains (cognitive, affective and psychomotor). It's important to mention that not all assessment instruments are suited for all children, because of their different disabilities. For that reason, modifications might be necessary to meet students' different needs, as well as to reach the desired expectations. The following sections will present examples of assessments for each learning domain. The priority of these domains is presented in no priority order.

Assessing the Psychomotor Domain

Teachers can measure the psychomotor domain by using existing or modified tools, or by creating their own assessment tools based on the program's goals and objectives. Instruments are available to assist with that task, regardless of the area in which the student is being assessed (e.g., safety, stroke development, water, sport games).

Figure 7.2 presents a modification of Texas Woman's University's Project Inspire Aquatic Assessment that teachers can use to determine a child's current performance level, as well as to document his/her progress. The original version of this instrument does not provide room to assess specific skills at two different times. Instead, it provides room only for teachers to indicate whether the skills are present or not.

Figure 7.2. Level 1 Aquatics Skill Assessment Checklist

Pre-Test		Child can:	Post-Test	
Yes	No		Yes	No
		Play with toys on the pool deck.		
		Sit on the edge of the pool with feet in the water and splash him/herself.		
		Sit on the edge of the pool and kick his/her feet in the water.		
		Climb down the pool ladder into chest-deep water.		
		Climb up the ladder to exit the pool.		
		Walk across the pool while holding onto the gutter.		
		Walk across the pool while holding the teacher's hand.		

— Adapted from "Adapted Aquatics for Individuals With Disabilities, Level 1," Project Inspire, Texas Woman's University. Used with permission.

Assessing students' ability with toys on a pool deck is important because, in some cases, students with disabilities might be afraid to enter the water. Playing with toys on the pool deck provides an excellent transition to introducing different equipment and exposing students to aquatic environments.

Figure 7.3 is another example of an aquatics assessment but involves swim strokes and is for children with higher swimming abilities. The teacher or peer should indicate whether the skills are present during both pre- and post-test.

Figure 7.3. Special Olympics Freestyle Checklist

Skill Progression – Freestyle

The Child Can:	Never	Sometimes	Often
Make an attempt to swim on front.			
Perform freestyle using flutter kick for 15 meters.			
Perform freestyle with rhythmic breathing for one pool length.			
Make an attempt to start, from in the pool.			
Perform proper start, standing on the pool edge.			
Perform proper start, using a starting block.			
Make an attempt to turn around without stopping.			
Perform an open turn after swimming freestyle without stopping.			
Perform a flip turn in waist-deep water.			
Perform flip turns after swimming one to two pool lengths.			

— Excerpted from *Special Olympics Aquatics Coaching Quick Start Guide* (2004). Used with permission.

When working in aquatic programs with a large numbers of students, teachers will benefit from the help of paraeducators, especially if some students have disabilities that can affect their performance in the pool. Therefore, it's important that teachers identify whether a student needs assistance to perform an activity and when the assistance is needed. Some students might need assistance for some of the activities, but not for all.

Figure 7.4 provides a way to identify the level of assistance a child might need to complete an activity.

Figure 7.4. Level 3 Aquatics Skills Assessment Checklist

Skill	N/A	P/A	T/A	Comments
Bob for 10 seconds.				
Bob for 20 seconds.				
Roll head to breathe and then blow bubbles, holding the gutter, 5 times in a row.				
Roll head to breathe and then blow bubbles, holding the gutter, 10 times in a row.				
Glide on stomach and recover to the feet.				

N/A = No assistance needed; P/A = Partial assistance needed; T/A = Total assistance needed

Note: The "Comments" section on this form can help teachers document student progress and keep information handy to support their findings when writing IEPs.

— Adapted from "Adapted Aquatics for Individuals With Disabilities, Level 3," Project Inspire, Texas Woman's University. Used with permission.

Assessing the Cognitive Domain

An cognitive test on aquatics should include items dealing with rules, equipment, techniques and strategies, among other aspects of swimming. Assessing children's performance levels in this area can aid the teacher's instruction and help students master skills beyond the aquatic environment, helping them maintain a healthy lifestyle. Depending on each child's cognitive level, the teacher can decide the best way to assess this domain.

If a child has only a physical disability and is able to take the same assessment as his/her peers, then that should be the choice. But if the child has any intellectual disability or is limited in communication abilities, the teacher must select an alternate strategy. Possible alternatives: an oral exam or using pictures so that the child can point to the correct answer. For example, if appropriate safety equipment is being taught, consider using this:

"What equipment do we use every time we enter the pool for a person who doesn't know how to swim?"

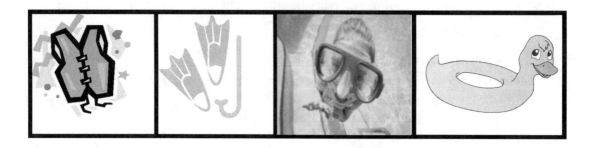

Two of those answers — the life jacket and the inflatable duck — can be correct; the desired correct answer will depend on which of the two the teacher has taught. If the child can't read, show the pictures and ask the question vocally.

Assessing the Affective Domain

The importance of assessing this domain can be explained for different reasons. First, students' attitudes toward physical activity — including aquatics — can determine how motivated they are to be physically active. Second, students have to interact with other students, which — depending on the disability — can involve some areas of the affective domain. (In addition, NASPE's *Moving Into the Future: National Standards for Physical Education* highlights the importance of teaching students social responsibility.)

Figures 7.5 and 7.6 can help teachers explore students' perceptions of their performance in the pool and their perceptions of how well they share with their peers.

Figure 7.5. Sample Student Perception Checklist

How much did you like working today in the pool?

… or …

How well did you share with your peers today during the activities?

1 Not at all —	2 Just a little -/+	3 It was okay +	4 Awesome ++

— Adapted from "Assessing the Cognitive and Affective Progress of Children," by Worrell, V., Evans-Fletcher, C. & Kovar, S., *Journal of Physical Education, Recreation and Dance,* 73 (7), 29-34. (2002), American Alliance for Health, Physical Education, Recreation and Dance.

Specific Modifications

Physical Disabilities

Transferring from the deck to the pool can be cumbersome for some children with physical disabilities. Therefore, teachers need to identify what type of device (e.g., chair, crutches, walker) that the child uses to move. Is the child able to transfer from the deck to the pool independently, or does he/she need assistance? Transfers are extremely important for children with physical disabilities. Assessing students' transfer abilities will inform staff and will promote students' move toward independence. Any program that is universally designed would include transfers as part of the assessment for aquatics, because it's part of the swimming process for some of the participants.

Figure 7.6. Deck-to-Pool Transfer Checklist

Yes	No	Skill	Comment
		The student communicates the best way of transferring.	
		The student is able to transfer on his/her own.	
		The student requires only one person to help with the transfer.	
		The student requires more than one person to help with the transfer.	

When assessing children with physical disabilities in aquatic environments, teachers need to keep three things in mind:

1. Watch the student's comfort level while in the water.

2. Pay attention to the student's range of motion and don't force the extremities.

3. Use a variety of equipment, including noodles and kick boards, to allow the student to rest between items.

Here are a few more suggested modifications:

- When assessing the stroke or kick of a swimmer with a physical disability, the teacher should follow the general rule that if a part of the body is absent or cannot be used, it is not assessed.

- Identify skills and body movements while watching others perform.

- Adjust routine to accommodate the child's ability (e.g., substitute upper-body movements for lower-body movements).

- Use the width of pool or lines to shorten distance.

- When assessing the kick, allow swimmers to hold onto a kickboard. If a student is unable to grip a kickboard, have him/her place a noodle or rescue tube underneath the armpits.

- When assessing the arm stroke, allow the child to use a pull buoy.

Cognitive, Communication & Autism Spectrum Disorders

Children with cognitive, communication and autism spectrum disorders will benefit from teachers' use of pictures, either during the assessment process or during instruction. Computer programs such as Boardmaker® can help facilitate that process for children who are nonverbal. Boardmaker® is a software program that uses clip art of picture communication symbols, which are used in creating printed communication boards, worksheets and schedules. Figure 7.7 presents a modification of the Texas Woman's University's Project Inspire Aquatic Assessment (Huettig, 1998) using Boardmaker®. *Note:* This is the same assessment tool as shown in Figure 7.2 but uses pictures.

Here are some more suggested modifications, adapted from *Adapted Aquatics Programming: A Professional Guide* (Human Kinetics, 2007) by Lepore, Gayle & Stevens:

- For children who are agitated easily, lead a relaxation activity before the assessment and emphasize self-control.

- To maximize understanding, keep instructions for the assessment brief.

- Repeat the assessment instructions and demonstrate the skill/stroke to be performed.

- Ask the student to repeat the instructions before the assessment begins.

Figure 7.7. Level I Aquatics Assessment Using Boardmaker®

HUETTIG'S ADAPTED AQUATICS ASSESSMENT

LEVEL 1

Students Name-_____

Date of Preliminary Evaluation-_____

I AM ABLE TO

YES	NO

PLAY WITH POOL TOYS   ON THE POOL DECK

SIT ON POOL EDGE WITH FEET IN THE POOL

SIT ON POOL EDGE WITH FEET IN THE POOL AND SPLASH MYSELF

I AM ABLE TO   LEVEL 1

YES	NO

SIT ON POOL EDGE WITH FEET IN THE POOL AND KICK MY FEET

CLIMB DOWN THE LADDER INTO THE POOL TO CHEST DEEP WATER

CLIMB UP THE LADDER TO GET OUT OF THE POOL

WALK ACROSS THE POOL HOLDING MY TEACHERS HAND

— Adapted from "Adapted Aquatics for Individuals With Disabilities, Level 1, Using Boardmaker®," Project Inspire, Texas Woman's University. Used with permission.

Emotional Disorders

Students with emotional disorders can have problems concentrating and remembering the sequencing of activities, so teachers might want to divide the assessment into two different sections of no more than 30 minutes each. That can help the student be more attentive to the instructions given. We also recommend that teachers offer a variety of activities that interest a child with emotional disorders, to maximize his/her chance of success. Administering a survey at the beginning of the sessions might help to identify the child's preferences.

Sensory Disorders

Vision

To maximize whatever available vision the student has:

- Wear a bright shirt and/or tights when demonstrating skill to be performed during assessment.

- Demonstrate the skill to be assessed directly in front of the students and no more than five to seven feet away.

- Keep assessment instructions concise.

- Use physical assistance when necessary.

Hearing

- Face the student and keep sentences short when giving assessment instructions to students who read lips.

- Use written or pictorial cue cards in combination with verbal assessment instructions.

- Use demonstrations as often as necessary.

We recommend the following books and online resources to further assist physical educators in teaching swimming to students with disabilities and developing an adapted aquatics program:

1. *Adapted Aquatics Programming: A Professional Guide* (Human Kinetics, 2007), by Lepore, Gayle & Stevens. An excellent resource, this book includes different assessment forms that teachers can modify to suit program needs, in addition to instruction considerations regarding adapted aquatics.

2. *Aquatic Readiness: Developing Water Competence in Young Children* (Human Kinetics, 1995), by Langendorfer & Bruya. Another good resource for teachers interested in developing a developmentally appropriate adapted aquatic program, this book provides assessment ideas and strategies to develop water competence in young children. Teachers can modify the activities presented in this book for children with disabilities.

3. Project Inspire, www.twu.edu/inspire/aquatics.asp. Developed by Texas Woman's University's Carol Huettig, this program provides not only ideas for physical activities for people with disabilities, but also provides advocacy, sports and adapted aquatics information.

Summary

The water is one of the most beneficial environments for students with disabilities. Especially for those with physical disabilities, the buoyancy of water helps students develop strength and endurance while allowing maximum mobility. With some creativity, patience and forethought, physical education teachers can modify their assessments to include all children in the class. This is the fundamental bases of UDL that ensures the opportunity for all children to benefit at the highest level from physical education class.

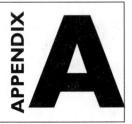

APPENDIX **A**

Glossary of Terms

Adapted physical education: A physical education program modified to meet the needs and abilities of students with disabilities.

Cognitive disability: Refers to a large spectrum of disorders and conditions, characterized by sub-average cognitive functioning. A person with cognitive disabilities has greater difficulty in one or more mental tasks than a "normal" or "average" person. Also, the person exhibits significant delays in measured intelligence, and adaptive and academic functioning (Needham, 2009). *Note:* also referred to as "intellectual disability."

Cerebral palsy: A condition involving damaged areas of the brain that impairs voluntary motor control or movement.

Inclusion: An education reform philosophy that promotes educating students with disabilities together with students without disabilities.

Individualized education program: A legal document developed to meet the education needs of a child with a disability by prescribing an appropriate plan for the child's education.

Orthotic device: An orthopedic brace or splint used to support, align, prevent or correct deformities or to improve the function of movable parts of the body.

Paraplegia: A neurological condition affecting movement of the legs but not the arms.

Picture schedules: Picture Exchange Communication System and Boardmaker® are two of several available visual-schedule software programs. Teachers can develop picture schedules and calendars with these programs and help facilitate the learning process for students who are non-verbal. Picture schedules often are developed for many students with autism because they help those children predict what will occur during the day or within the class.

Quadriplegia: A neurological condition that impairs movement of all four limbs.

Spina bifida: An incomplete closure of the vertebral arch(es) of the spinal column. The most severe form can result in partial to complete impairment of mobility in the lower limbs.

Visual impairment: A significant limitation or loss of vision resulting from disease, trauma or congenital or degenerative conditions that cannot be corrected.

References

Apache, R.R., Hisey, P. & Blanchard, L. (2005). An adapted aquatics assessment inventory and curriculum. *Palaestra, 21,* 32-37.

Baker, D. (2001). *Elementary heart health: Lessons and assessment.* Reston, VA: National Association for Sport and Physical Education.

Block, M.E., Lieberman, L.J., & Conner-Kuntz, F. (1998). Authentic assessment in adapted physical education, *Journal of Physical Education, Recreation and Dance, 69*(3), 48-56.

Borg, G. (1998) *Borg's perceived exertion and pain scales.* Champaign, IL: Human Kinetics.

Boswell, B. (2005). Adapted rhythms and dance. In J.P. Winnick (Ed.) *Adapted physical education and sport.* Champaign, IL: Human Kinetics.

Bowerman, S. (2007). *Assessment in adapted aquatics.* Project Inspire. Texas Woman's University. Retrieved June 28, 2010, from www.twu.edu/inspire/aquatics.asp.

Cone, T. & Cone, S. (2005). *Assessing dance in elementary physical education.* Reston, VA: National Association for Sport and Physical Education.

Davis, R. (2002). *Inclusion through sport.* Champaign, IL: Human Kinetics.

Ellis, K., Lieberman, L.J. & Leroux, D. (2009). Using differentiated instruction in physical education, *Palaestra, 24,* 19-23.

Foley, J., Harvey, S., Hae-Ja, C. & So-Yeun, K. (2008). The relationships among fundamental motor skills, health-related physical fitness and body fatness in South Korean adolescents with mental retardation. *Research Quarterly for Exercise & Sport, 79*(2), 149-157.

Foley, J., Tindall, D.W., Lieberman, L.J. & Kim, S. (2007). How to develop disability awareness using the Sport Education Model. *The Journal of Physical Education, Recreation and Dance, 78,* 32-36.

Gross, S. J. (2005). *Assessment of swimming in physical education.* Reston, VA: National Association for Sport and Physical Education.

Holt/Hale, S. (1999) *Assessing motor skills in elementary physical education.* Reston, VA: National Association for Sport and Physical Education.

Holt/Hale, S. (1999). *Assessing and improving fitness in elementary physical education.* Reston, VA: National Association for Sport and Physical Education.

Houston-Wilson, C. (2005). Pervasive developmental disorders. In J. P. Winnick (Ed.) *Adapted physical education and sport.* Champaign, IL: Human Kinetics.

Huettig, C. (1998). Texas Woman's University aquatic skills assessment. Retrieved August 7, 2008, from www.twu.edu/inspire/aquatics.asp.

Huettig, C. & Darden-Melton, B. (2004). Acquisition of aquatic skills by children with autism. *Palaestra (20)*2, 20- 27.

Humphries, K.M. (2008). Humphries' Assessment of Aquatic Readiness (HAAR). Project Inspire. Texas Woman's University. Retrieved June 28, 2010, from www.twu.edu/inspire/aquatics.asp.

Kaufmann, K. (2006). *Inclusive creative movement and dance.* Champaign, IL: Human Kinetics.

Kelly, L. (2011). Spinal cord disabilities. In J.P. Winnick (Ed.) *Adapted physical education and sport.* Champaign, IL: Human Kinetics.

Kowalski, E. (2000). Adapted rhythms and dance. In J. Winnick (Ed.) *Adapted physical education and sport* (3rd ed.). Champaign, IL: Human Kinetics.

Kowalski, E., Houston-Wilson, C., Daggett, S., Speedling, R. & Douglas, B. (Under contract). *Inclusive physical education assessment: From basic to proficiency.* Champaign, IL: Human Kinetics.

Langendorfer, S.J., & Bruya, L.D. (1995). *Aquatic readiness: Developing water competence in young children.* Champaign, IL: Human Kinetics.

Lepore, M., Gayle, G.W. & Stevens, S. (2007). *Adapted aquatics programming: A professional guide.* Champaign, IL: Human Kinetics.

Leroux, D., Lieberman, L.J. & Ellis, K. (In press). Using differentiated instruction in physical education. *Palaestra.*

Lieberman, L.J. (2002). Fitness for individuals who are visually impaired or deaf blind. *Review* Spring 34 (1) 13.

Lieberman, L.J. (2011). Visual impairments. In J. P. Winnick (Ed.) *Adapted physical education and sport,* (5th edition). Champaign, IL: Human Kinetics.

Lieberman, L.J. (2007) (Ed.). *Paraeducators in physical education.* Champaign, IL: Human Kinetics.

Lieberman, L.J., & Houston-Wilson, C. (2009). *Strategies for inclusion; A handbook for physical educators,* (2nd ed.). Champaign, IL: Human Kinetics.

Lieberman, L.J., Lytle, R.K., & Clarq, J.A. (2008). Getting it right from the start: Employing the Universal Design for Learning approach to your curriculum, *Journal of Physical Education, Recreation and Dance, 79,* 32-39.

Lockette, K., & Keyes, A. (1994). *Conditioning with physical disabilities.* Champaign, IL: Human Kinetics.

Lund, J. L. (2000). *Creating rubrics for physical education.* Reston, VA: National Association for Sport and Physical Education.

Meredith, M. & Welk, G. (1999). *Fitnessgram: Test administration manual,* (2nd ed.). Champaign, IL: Human Kinetics.

Meyer, A. & Rose, D.H. (2000). Universal design for individual differences. *Educational Leadership, 58*(3), 39-43.

Mitchell, S.A. & Oslin, J.L. (1999). *Assessment in games teaching*. Reston, VA: National Association for Sport and Physical Education.

National Association for Sport and Physical Education (2005). *Physical Best activity guide: Elementary level, (2nd ed.)*. Champaign, IL: Human Kinetics.

Odem, S. L., Brantlinger, E., Gersten, R., R.H., Thompson, B. & Harris, K.R. (2005). Research in special education: Scientific methods and evidence-based practices. *Exceptional Children, 71*, 137-148.

Physical activity and fitness for persons with disabilities. *PCPFS research digest.*

Rink, J. (2009). *Teaching physical education for learning, (6th ed.).* St. Louis: Mosby.

Rose, D. H. & Meyer, A. (2002). *Teaching every student in the digital age: Universal design for learning*. Alexandria, VA: Association for Supervision and Curriculum Development.

Rowland, T. (2005). *Children's exercise physiology, (2nd ed.)*. Champaign, IL: Human Kinetics.

Schiemer, S. (2000). *Assessment strategies for elementary physical education*. Champaign, IL: Human Kinetics.

Short, F. (2005). Health-related physical fitness and physical activity. In Winnick, Joseph P. (ed.), *Adapted physical education and Sport,* (4th ed.). Champaign, IL: Human Kinetics.

Special Olympics (2004). Special Olympics aquatics coaching quick start guide. Retrieved June 28, 2010, from www.specialolympics.org.

Sugden, D. & Keogh, J. (1990). *Problems in movement skill development*. Columbia, SC: University of South Carolina Press.

Thousand, S.J., Villa, R.A. & Nevin, A.I. (2007). *Differentiating instruction*. Thousand Oaks, CA: Corwin Press.

Tripp, A., Rizzo, T. & Webbert, L. (2007). Inclusion in physical education: Changing the culture. *Journal of Physical Education, Recreation and Dance*. 78(2), 34.

Ulrich, D.A. (2000). *The test of gross motor development*. Austin, TX: Pro-Ed.

Winnick, J., & Short, F. (2005). Conceptual framework for the Brockport physical fitness test. *Adapted Physical Activity Quarterly, 22* (1) 323-332.

Winnick, J. & Short, F. (2005). Introduction to the Brockport physical fitness test technical manual. *Adapted Physical Activity Quarterly, 22* (1) 315-322.

Winnick, J. & Short, F. (2005) Test items and standards related to aerobic functioning on the Brockport physical fitness test. *Adapted Physical Activity Quarterly, 22* (1), 333-355.

Winnick, J. & Short, F. (2005). Test items and standards related to the muscular strength and endurance on the Brockport physical fitness test. *Adapted Physical Activity Quarterly, 22* (1) 371-400.

Winnick, J. & Short, F. (1999). *The Brockport physical fitness test manual*. Champaign, IL. Human Kinetics.

Worrell, V., Evans-Fletcher, C. & Kovar, S. (2002). Assessing the cognitive and affective domain progress of children. *Journal of Physical Education, Recreation and Dance, 73(7)*, 28-34.

Resources

Published by the National Association for Sport and Physical Education:

PE Metrics: Assessing National Standards 1 – 6 in Secondary School (2011)
The Physical Educator's Guide to Successful Grant Writing, 2nd Edition (2011)
PE Metrics: Assessing National Standards 1 – 6 in Elementary School (2010)
Concepts and Principles of Physical Education: What Every Student Should Know, 3rd Edition (2010)
Physical Activity and Sport for the Secondary School Student, 6th Edition (2010)
Principles of Safety in Physical Education and Sport, 4th Edition (2010)
National Standards & Guidelines for Physical Education Teacher Education (2009)
Active Start: A Statement of Physical Activity Guidelines for Children From Birth to Age 5, 2nd Edition (2009)
Never Play Leapfrog With a Unicorn: K – 5 Physical Activities to Meet the Standards (2007)
Movement-Based Learning: Academic Concepts & Physical Activity for Children Ages 3 – 8 (2007)
Quality Coaches, Quality Sports: National Standards for Sport Coaches (2006)
Moving Into the Future: National Standards for Physical Education, 2nd Edition (2004)

Assessment Series

Assessing and Improving Fitness in Elementary Physical Education, 2nd Edition (2008)
Standards-Based Assessment of Student Learning: A Comprehensive Approach, 2nd Edition (2007)
Assessing Dance in Elementary Physical Education (2005)
Assessment of Swimming in Phyical Education (2005)
Assessing Concepts: Secondary Biomechanics (2004)
Assessing Student Outcomes in Sport Education (2003)
Assessment in Outdoor Adventure Physical Education (2003)
Assessing Heart Rate in Physical Education (2002)
Authentic Assessment of Physical Activity for High School Students (2002)
Elementary Heart Health: Lessons and Assessment (2001)
Creating Rubrics for Physical Education (2000)
Assessing Motor Skills in Elementary Physical Education (1999)
Assessment in Games Teaching (1999)

Order online at www.aahperd.org/shop or call (800) 321-0789

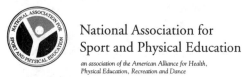

National Association for
Sport and Physical Education
an association of the American Alliance for Health, Physical Education, Recreation and Dance

NASPE Sets the Standard

1900 Association Drive • Reston, Va. 20191
703-476-3400 • 703-476-8316 (fax)
www.naspeinfo.org